Biofeedback and
Family Practice
Medicine

Biofeedback and Family Practice Medicine

Edited by
William H. Rickles
Sepulveda Veterans Administration Hospital
The School of Medicine, UCLA
Los Angeles, California

Jack H. Sandweiss
Sandweiss Biofeedback Institute
Beverly Hills, California

David W. Jacobs
Biofeedback Institute of San Diego
San Diego, California

Robert N. Grove
United States International University
San Diego, California

and
Eleanor Criswell
Sonoma State University
Rohnert, California

PLENUM PRESS • NEW YORK AND LONDON

Library of Congress Cataloging in Publication Data

Conference on Biofeedback and Family Practice Medicine (1980: San Jose, Calif.)
   Biofeedback and family practice medicine.

   "Based on a Conference on Biofeedback and Family Practice Medicine, cosponsored by the Biofeedback Society of California, the Department of Continuing Education and Health Sciences, UCLA Extension, and The School of Medicine, UCLA, held
November 13–15, 1980, at the Annual Biofeedback Society of California Meeting,
in San Jose, California"—T.p. verso.
   Includes bibliographical references and index.
   1. Medicine, Psychosomatic—Congresses. 2. Biofeedback training—Congresses.
3. Family medicine—Congresses. I. Rickles, William H. II. Biofeedback Society of
California. III. Title. [DNLM: 1. Biofeedback (Psychology)—Congresses. 2. Family
practice—Congresses. WL 103 C748b 1980]
RC49.C59 1980   616.08   83-11111
ISBN 0-306-41386-8

Based on a Conference on Biofeedback and Family Practice Medicine,
cosponsored by the Biofeedback Society of California, the Department of
Continuing Education and Health Sciences, UCLA Extension, and The School of
Medicine, UCLA, held November 13–15, 1980, at the Annual Biofeedback
Society of California Meeting, in San Jose, California

© 1983 Plenum Press, New York
A Division of Plenum Publishing Corporation
233 Spring Street, New York, N.Y. 10013

PREFACE

During the past five years there has been a reawakening of
interest in the psychotherapy of patients with medical disorders
characterized as psychosomatic. For three decades, psychoanalysis
and psychoanalytic psychotherapy were used extensively to treat and
study psychosomatic disorders. Early in the 1960s, interest in
this approach to these conditions faded, and the "Psychosomatic
Service" in most hospitals became the "Consultation Liaison Service"
(Lipowski, 1967). The recent focus of biofeedback on psychosomatic
conditions provides a new technique with which the physician or
psychiatrist may treat these patients (Rickles, 1981).

In addition, the successful application of biofeedback training
to a variety of complaints such as those presented in this volume
has heralded the addition of biofeedback to the treatment modalities
used for medical complaints. Frequently, psychological factors can
still be seen; for example, when biofeedback treatment may require
lifestyle changes on the part of the patient, the exploration of
secondary gains or resistances before the disorder can be successfully treated, and the establishment of rapport and empathy which is
so important for truly effective biofeedback training. Aside from
certain psychological dimensions that are always present in biofeedback training, in this case biofeedback is being used in a primarily
medical setting for primarily medical complaints.

Biofeedback involves the use of electronic devices to measure
physiological function, with the data from that measurement fed back
to the patient in the form of lights, sounds or quantities. The
information fed back to the patient enables him to alter the physiological function being recorded. With biofeedback training, alteration of the function is increasingly in the desired direction. For
example, a decrease in muscle tone has been associated with successful management of tension headaches in some cases. Biofeedback has
shown itself solidly efficacious in the laboratory and in clinical
studies for a number of presenting complaints. Furthermore, it has
additional contributions to make to family care medicine because of

the shift that it makes in patient responsibility--the return of the
doctor/patient relationship to a shared responsibility. The result
of biofeedback is increased cooperation of the patient in the course
of treatment. The effectiveness of biofeedback for certain complaints and the relative lack of negative side effects of biofeedback treatment are two of its most valuable contributions to family
practice medicine.

In November, 1979, William H. Rickles, M.D., was named by David
Jacobs, incoming President of the Biofeedback Society of California,
as Program Chairman of the 1980 BSC Annual Convention. Jack
Sandweiss and Robert N. Grove soon joined him as co-chairmen of the
Program Committee. At that time, the idea of doing a specialized
symposium co-sponsored with UCLA Extension in conjunction with the
BSC Annual Convention emerged. It seemed that it was time to highlight the clinical and laboratory research which supported the use
of biofeedback in conjunction with medical care as the treatment of
choice for a variety of presenting complaints. At that time, it was
also determined that an edited volume of the symposium presentations
would be worthwhile. The symposium and subsequent book were to be
titled: Biofeedback and Family Practice Medicine. The symposium
was held in San Jose, California; presenters were flown in from
various locations in California and other parts of the United States.
Participants from a variety of professions attended: physicians,
psychiatrists, nurses, physical therapists, psychologists, occupational therapists, social workers, educators, and others. The
result was an excellent collection of presentations and discussions
fully expressing the state of the art in the interface between biofeedback and family or primary practice medicine--topics, viewpoints,
information, issues.

This book is designed for the family care or primary care physician desiring information in order to make appropriate referrals
for biofeedback when it is indicated by the nature of the presenting
complaint. It is also useful for those wanting to respond appropriately to their patients who, having heard about biofeedback,
request a biofeedback referral for a particular complaint. Psychiatrists, nurses, physical therapists, psychologists, and other health
care providers who serve as referral sources for biofeedback from
family practice physicians, will also find it useful.

Increasingly, insurance companies are reimbursing for biofeedback training when biofeedback is indicated, i.e., when other established treatment procedures have been tried unsuccessfully and/or
when the case warrants the use of biofeedback based on clinical and
laboratory biofeedback research. Reimbursement is based on physician diagnosis. This requires that the physician be aware of when
biofeedback would be indicated, where in the series of proscribed

procedures it might best fit, and when it would be used in combination with other treatments such as in a multimodality approach.

This book is designed for those who are interested in the
application of biofeedback to problems of family and primary practice medicine. Therefore, our emphasis has been on some of the common complaints seen by the family practice physician and how they
have been treated by clinical and laboratory biofeedback. The
articles in this book are the work of innovative clinician/research-
ers who are solidly experienced in the field of clinical biofeedback
and their areas of expertise. The format of the articles is variable. Some of them include information about the presenting complaint and how biofeedback has been used in treating it. Others
also include examples of treatment procedures. The list of medical
complaints and issues addressed by this book includes: hypertension,
pulmonary disorders, headaches, physical medicine problems, fecal
incontinence, problems of children, dermatological complaints,
Raynaud's diathesis, personality characteristics of psychosomatic
patients, and many others. Discussion sections follow many of the
articles. The approach to these treatment areas sometimes indicates
biofeedback as the treatment of choice or the multimodality use of
biofeedback. In some cases, it is clear that biofeedback would not
be indicated. It is important to know clearly when biofeedback is
or is not appropriate.

In conclusion, biofeedback is becoming the treatment of choice
for a variety of complaints. Some family or primary practice physicians are incorporating biofeedback into their practices; others are
making referrals to other practitioners when biofeedback is indicated. The main aim of this book is to supply the information
necessary for the family practice physician and other health care
providers to make appropriate treatment and referral choices.

The editors of this volume would like to thank the Biofeedback
Society of California and the Department of Continuing Education in
Health Sciences, UCLA Extension, and The School of Medicine, UCLA
for producing the Biofeedback and Family Practice symposium, and the
symposium participants for making a thorough exploration of these
topics. We wish to thank the contributors to the volume. We would
also like to thank the following: Ronald L. Linder, UCLA Extension,
Continuing Education in Health Sciences, Susanne Oliver, who served
as Program Coordinator for the symposium; Cognetics, for their
excellent recordings of the symposium; Allegra Broughton, who typed
portions of the manuscript; Deena Spikell and her staff at Letter
Perfect, Los Angeles, for their word processing services which helped
the volume move toward the level of perfection that it required;
Marsha Calhoun, for assistance in copy editing; Artur Argrewicz,
Dorothy Alegre, Michael Baron, Diana Brewer, Halimah Cristy, Vici
Froland, Randy Lefevre, Laura Katzman, Wesley Hiler, Gordon

Matheless, Carl Michels, Mar Putterman, Geoff Ranch-Apple, Joie
Sequeira, and Regina Williams, who helped prepare the index; and Pat
Vann at Plenum, for her patience, understanding and firmness.

                                    William H. Rickles
                                    Jack H. Sandweiss
                                    David Jacobs
                                    Robert N. Grove
                                    Eleanor Criswell

                                    Los Angeles, California
                                    Summer, 1982

REFERENCES

Lipowski, Z. J. Review of consultation psychiatry and psychosomatic
      medicine. II. Clinical aspects. Psychosomatic Medicine, 1967,
      29, 201-224.

Rickles, W. H. Biofeedback Therapy and transitional phenomena.
      Psychiatric Annals, 1981.

CONTENTS

BIOFEEDBACK: A PARADIGM FOR THE SELF-REGULATION OF HEALTH CARE

David W. Jacobs

Director, Biofeedback Institute of San Diego
San Diego, California

The publication of reports in the 1960s concerning self-regulated physiological control led to much speculation about the advantages to be gained from biofeedback. It was an unfortunate time for serious researchers in the field. "Alpha" parlors sprang up around the country promising enhanced creativity, greater sexual awareness and other untold benefits. It was a number of years before these gimmicky aspects of biofeedback faded from public consciousness, but we have now reached the point where it is possible to consider, in a sober and careful way, the potential value of biofeedback for health care. The papers that follow will demonstrate this perspective in detail.

My purpose is to provide a theoretical analysis of this field in two areas. The first is a conceptual model of what biofeedback is and why it works when it does. The second is to examine some of the broader implications of biofeedback for health care.

We will begin this process by presenting a case history to illustrate how biofeedback is typically used in a clinical setting. The information will be used as a touchstone against which to examine the process called biofeedback.

This is the case of Mr. T., a 28 year old Caucasian male employed as an engineer in a local electronics firm. He was referred to the Biofeedback Institute of San Diego by a neurologist who had completed an examination after referral from the family physician. The chief complaint was daily chronic pain in a band-like area at the approximate level of the frontal muscles extending from the occiput to the forehead. Associated with this was soreness and occasional pain in the upper insertions of the trapezius and

sterno-mastoid muscles. This pain was described as at its low point
during the morning, increasing toward the late afternoon and at its
worst between 4:00 and 6:00 p.m. The overall pain pattern was typically reduced on weekends.

The patient had suffered from this problem for approximately
three years prior to the time of seeing the neurologist. The
problem had grown worse, starting with occasional headaches which
gradually increased in intensity, frequency, and duration. His
prior medical history was unremarkable, except for having had the
measles and mumps as a child. There is no history of headache
problems among members of his immediate family. The findings of
both his physician and neurologist were negative, although the
neurologist in his referring report indicated a certain amount of
soreness and tenderness in the upper insertions of the trapezius
muscles upon palpation.

This patient had been on an increasing regimen of medication
for headaches during the three year period of the difficulty. He
reported that the head pain had been responsive to aspirin in the
early stages, but that this had become decreasingly effective and
was replaced with medications like Darvocet, Empirin, and, when the
head pain was unusually bad, Empirin with codeine.

His social history was rather conventional. The patient was
married at the age of 24, after graduation from college, and has two
children. He characterized his marriage as uneventful, if somewhat
boring. He was sexually active with his wife and characterized his
sex life as satisfactory. Some significant difficulties, however,
were indicated with regard to his work. The industry in which he
works is a highly competitive one and he was subject to many
pressures from his supervisors. He found going to work increasingly
distasteful and had, in the last year, begun to take time off from
work because of his head pain. He reported that for the first time
in his life he had begun to question his career choice. In his
relations with peers he spontaneously offered a description of himself as a "loner," with no friends and few acquaintances. His only
hobby was photography, which he typically indulged in by himself.
He had no regular forms of exercise, although reporting that occasionally he and his wife played tennis together on Sunday mornings.

Initial myographic measurements from the frontal muscles were
made with surface electrodes and filters set at 100-600 Hz. The
readings during a 20-minute period with the subject in a semi-
reclined position averaged 18 microvolts, about double the expected
readings for a normal person. In the absence of other significant
findings, a tentative diagnosis of chronic muscle contraction headaches was made, which was in concurrence with the diagnosis of both
his family physician and the neurologist.

This patient was given a course of 10 biofeedback treatments for his condition. The treatments consisted of approximately 40 minutes each on a weekly basis, during which time the patient was seated in a semi-reclined position in a chair. Surface electrodes with the myograph were placed on the frontalis muscles and the resulting muscle activity was displayed on the meter in view of the patient. Mr. T. was asked to reduce the muscle tension displayed on the meter. During this time, Mr. T. discovered that the tension and pain in his forehead resulted from chronic contractions of the masseter, sternomastoid, and trapezius musceles and that deliberate relaxation of these muscles produced a reduction in tension and pain. He was, in addition, provided with cassette tapes of muscle relaxation instructions for daily use at home and was put on a program of daily exercise.

Mr. T.'s condition improved steadily during the course of treatment. Average muscle readings for the periods of time in therapy dropped from baseline to 7.5 microvolts at the last treatment session. Mr. T. had also been asked to rate average head pain per day and to record the amount of medication taken. While he faithfully kept records during the first several weeks and he recorded precipitant drops in average pain and medication taken, Mr. T. grew increasingly disinterested in maintaining these records, which are therefore not available for the whole period of treatment. However, by the final session he reported that he had had only one headache in the prior week, immediately following an argument with his wife. He had taken no medication during that period of time. Mr. T. was seen once more four weeks after the last session for an initial follow-up. At that time, his average muscle tension ratings were 8.4 microvolts. He reported that there had only been one or two headaches in the intervening month, both of which he successfully aborted with muscle relaxation techniques. The final contact with Mr. T. was made 90 days after the one month follow-up. He reported that he had a short period of time, approximately six weeks after the termination of therapy, when he had had headaches for several days, but there had been no head pain since then. There has been no subsequent follow-up.

Case reports of this type usually arouse several emotions in the medically trained listener. The first is a feeling of incredulity. Here is a patient suffering from chronic head pain, treated by well-trained medical personnel, but with a steady increase in severity of symptoms. Yet the simple act of sitting in front of a myograph and watching changes in its meter output produces a rapid change in pain and the physiological conditions subsuming it. The typical reaction might be to dismiss the treatment as a placebo, but if the term placebo implies changes in psychological condition which are not accompanied by corresponding changes in physiological condition, this case does not meet the definition. Very real, substantive changes in physiological state were produced by this apparently innocuous act.

The other reaction which is normally engendered in almost any
listener, whether medically trained or not, is an intuitive feeling
of correctness about the training procedure. There is something
about disorders like muscle contraction headaches which implies
that, somehow or other, the patient has brought the disease on himself and that it is therefore within his power to cure it. Patients
suffering from muscle contraction head pain often report such a
view. Phrases like, "If I could only relax" and "I wish I could
make this go away" are frequently heard. They imply an awareness
that this disorder seems to them susceptible to self-control. Yet
there is also the undeniable fact that the disorder is not self-
controlled, that bodily activities are not altered in such a way as
to produce a cure. It seems that some change needs to occur in the
functioning of these patients before self-regulation is possible.
In some sense, then, the biofeedback training acts as a precipitant
or catalyst in the development of such a change. It is with this
notion and an extended model of it that the next section of this
paper will be concerned.

SELF-REGULATED BEHAVIOR: A CYBERNETICS APPROACH

One way of understanding Mr. T.'s cure is to define it as an
exercise in self-regulation. In place of the chronic tension Mr.
T. experienced in the muscles of his head, neck and shoulders, he
learned to induce deliberately a state of relaxation in those
muscles by regulating the tension levels. If this is typical of the
way in which biofeedback works (and the case was selected because of
its typicalness), what are the conditions under which this self-
regulation takes place? A simple demonstration may suffice to
illustrate those conditions.

Consider an experiment in which a subject is seated in front
of a table, his arm extended, with a curtain between his hand and
the rest of his arm. The experimental task is to draw lines 2 cm.
long on a pad. From the perspective of increasing the self-
regulation of his behavior, consider various consequences which may
follow each attempt to draw a line. These are given in Table 1,
which is arranged in order of increasing knowledge of results. The

Table 1. Conditions of Feedback in a
Line-Drawing Experiment

No Feedback
Binary Feedback
Tertiary Feedback
Quantitative Feedback
Unrestricted Feedback

first is labeled the no-feedback consequence. After the subject
draws a line, he is simply instructed to draw another line. In the
second condition, labeled binary feedback, the subject is only told
whether the line was of the correct length or not. In tertiary
feedback, the subject is told either that the line was too long, too
short, or of the correct length. In quantitative feedback, the subject is told the actual length of the line drawn on each trial. In
the final condition, the curtain is removed and the subject sees his
own performance relative to some standard line.

   The prediction, clearly, is that the subject's performance
would be enhanced with each increment of completeness of feedback,
and the implications are clear. Knowledge of results about one's
own performance makes possible a rapid and effective change in that
performance. Turning back to the case of Mr. T., one can argue that
the reason biofeedback training helped was that he was placed in a
loop similar to the one created by one of the levels of feedback in
the line drawing study. By constantly feeding back information
about the state of his musculature, he was able to learn to self-
regulate it in the same way as did the subject in the line drawing
study.

   It is now possible to provide a definition of biofeedback.
Biofeedback is a procedure in which physiological output from an
organism is fed back as input to that organism as an aid in the
self-regulation of that output. Our problem is to understand why
this should occur.

   One model for understanding why biofeedback works arises from
the field of cybernetics. The term "cybernetics" is derived from an
ancient Greek word referring to the steersman or helmsman of a boat
(Weiner, 1948). The discipline is concerned with the ways in which
systems are regulated, i.e., prevented from going out of control.
This is what a helmsman does on a boat. By making small adjustments
in the tiller, which produce larger adjustments in the position of
the rudder, still larger changes are made in the direction of the
boat's forward movement. The movements of the helmsman are compen-
sations for changes in wind and water conditions. If the movement
of the boat was taken as the output and viewed from a vantage point
above the boat, the boat would not be seen as traveling in a
straight line, but as traveling in a series of small zig-zag movements around a straight line which defined its true course.

   Comparable analyses can be made of many other systems.
Consider the operation of a governor on a steam boiler. When the
boiler reaches a critical point, a valve opens, steam escapes, and
the pressure in the boiler drops to some lower level. The valve
then closes and the pressure begins to build in the boiler again.
As is the case with the course of a boat, the pressure in the boiler
varies around some optimal pre-set figure. At any one point in

time, the pressure will be determined by the actions of the valve
vis-a-vis the internal pressure of the boiler.

We now have three examples of systems under control: the behavior of a subject in an experiment drawing lines; the behavior of
a boat; and the behavior of a steam boiler. The genius of Weiner's
analysis lies in the fact that comparable characteristics can be
discussed in all three systems. For example, in any one of them,
control disappears if the output of the system is not permitted to
feed back to the system. In the first case, line drawing, there
would not be any particular change in the length of the lines drawn.
In the second, the boat would drift off course, subject to the
vagaries of wind and current. In the last case, the steam boiler
would explode. Control only becomes available when the output of
the system loops back so that it alters the input of the system in
some regular fashion. The feedback sets the stage for the control.

Weiner does point out, however, that there are two possible
ways in which feedback can produce effects. One of these, positive
feedback, has the output of the system looping back into the system
to accelerate its performance, i.e., it accentuates the ongoing
change. This phenomenon produces loss of control, as can be illustrated in the behavior of profoundly stressed patients. Their
history frequently starts as a moderate stress state, which produces
a limited degree of withdrawal from social contact and enjoyable
activities. Such withdrawal usually increases the amount of stress
the patient feels, which accelerates the withdrawal, which in turn
accelerates the feelings of stress and depression. This positive
feedback loop, if unchecked, can result in chronic severe
depression.

The other alternative is the negative feedback loop described
above, in which the output of the system is used to moderate the
input and produce a steady state within the system. It is this
latter condition, negative feedback, which makes possible the self-
regulation of any system.

CYBERNETICS, SELF-REGULATION AND HEALTH CARE

Given this theoretical notion, it is possible to ask how organ-
isms physiologically maintain themselves in a healthy state. From
a cybernetic point of view, an excellent example of a health care
strategy derives from the concept of homeostasis. As originally
developed by Cannon (1932), the notion stated that there were certain mechanisms in the body which controlled its internal state in a
steady state form. These mechanisms of self-regulation are designed
to maintain a constant internal state in spite of variations in the
external environment, primarily through the activity of the autonomic nervous system (ANS). The ANS modulates the activity of the

(visceral) organ systems relative to the needs of the body. Negative feedback loops exist within the ANS to maintain visceral activity within narrow limits. Examples of this type of self-regulation can be found in the control of such activities as internal temperature, arterial blood pressure, gastric pH and heart rate.

What makes all of this so interesting is that all of these complex activities are carried on automatically. The control requires no conscious effort and no input from the external environment. This automaticity is what makes homeostatic mechanisms so important as a health care strategy. The system is morphologically and physiologically structured to provide a healthy state of the organism, unless seriously interfered with from the outside.

But these mechanisms of homeostatic control are contained within the framework of the total organism. For this larger system, questions may be raised about what types of self-regulation are available where there is no homeostatic control, e.g., in those behaviors modulated by the central nervous system (CNS).

One alternative is to define self-regulation as a skill to be learned through a series of specific steps. Such learning is difficult because the negative feedback loops in the CNS do not operate in an automatic fashion, as in the ANS. The CNS functions to permit many more possible behaviors than the ANS. Which ones are realized depends on the environmental contingencies. For such health-related activities as exercise and diet, there are few naturally occurring feedback loops to provide control. Some other form of intervention may therefore be necessary so that the patient can learn the appropriate forms of self-regulation.

While not all aspects of self-regulation are known, several can be defined. Perhaps the most important of these is the development of behavior patterns which are alternatives to the ones that are already learned. It is a good maxim in behavioral work of any kind that no behavior disappears, it is simply replaced by an alternative behavior. Certainly this is the case with the self-regulation of behavior patterns related to health. Examples of this abound in the literature dealing with the treatment of addictive disorders. Alcohol abusers, for example, are frequently faced with the problem of deciding what to do if they are not to be occupied with drinking behavior. A significant portion of therapy for such patients involves the development of alternative patterns of behavior. Sometimes these behavior patterns need to be quite precisely shaped. Recovering alcoholics frequently need to be trained into a ritualized pattern for refusing the offer of an alcoholic drink, simply because they do not know how to refuse one in a manner they would regard as acceptable. It is important, then, that specific behavior patterns relevant to optimal health be trained in the development of self-regulation.

Concomitant with this is the development of appropriate cognitive and emotional states. As Ellis (1976) has often pointed out,
the emotional and belief components involved with any behavior pattern must be consistent with the behavior in order to sustain it.
For example, a patient learning to manage a drinking problem may
have great difficulty sustaining abstinence if he does not also
learn to feed back his successes in averting a period of drinking.
Such apparently minor changes in cognitive control are critical in
the development and maintenance of self-regulated behaviors. This
point will be amplified in a subsequent section of this paper.

The point to be emphasized here is that self-regulation consists primarily of a series of small steps such as those described
above, which, when taken together, form a coherent and stable pattern of behavior. One cannot simply decide to self-regulate a
health related behavior any more than one can simply decide to ride
a bicycle. The steps necessary to acquire the skill must be gone
through. There are a number of reasons why learning to behave in a
self-regulated fashion is difficult when there is no homeostatic
control. Perhaps the most obvious of these is that the patterns
which are non-self-regulatory have a long history for the organism
and are therefore deeply habituated. In working with individuals
for self-regulated change, one frequently encounters childhood
events which set the stage for the current difficulty. A most
obvious example of this is found in childhood patterns of maladaptive eating behaviors in which more food than could possibly be
justified by caloric outgo was urged upon a child as a routine
matter. In such an environment, overeating becomes a habitual pattern and is therefore highly resistant to change. The second reason
why the patterns of adaptive self-regulation are hard to initiate is
that the older patterns are frequently highly reinforcing. The
physiological sequelae of cigarette smoking are noxious to the
novice smoker, but to the experienced smoker they represent a source
of profound satisfaction and tension reduction. Such reinforcement
carries with it a strong resistance to changing behavior patterns
which, at least at their initiation, may not be nearly as satis-
fying. Finally, there is a great deal of support in this society
for certain maladaptive behavior patterns. Both cigarette smoking
and overeating are none too subtly encouraged by the media or
modeled by large numbers of people in our everyday environments and
are frequently the subject of direct social approval. Examples of
this effect are so common for eating, drinking, and smoking that
documentation is not necessary.

BIOFEEDBACK IN THE REGULATION OF MALADAPTIVE BEHAVIORS

From a cybernetic point of view, biofeedback is an exterior
negative feedback loop running parallel to the body's own negative
feedback loop. By providing an external loop, information that it

doesn't otherwise have is made available. One of the difficulties involved in gaining control of visceral behaviors is that they represent "silent" processes in the body, i.e., they provide no conscious information about the state of the organ system. By providing that information, biofeedback makes feasible the possibility of such control. As some of the papers in this volume suggest, where the negative feedback loop is available, control is often achievable. Indeed, it may be the case that the only limit on control of these functions will be imposed by the limits of technology to make these silent processes signal bearing. This model holds particularly well in activities controlled by the ANS.

For example, biofeedback has demonstrated its use in the control of peripheral vasomotor activity in Raynaud's syndrome. In this disease, vasospasms are typically initiated by cold temperature, some emotional stressor or physical trauma. Biofeedback treatment for this disorder consists of placing the patient in a negative feedback loop with an electronic thermometer, the sensor of which is placed on one of the affected digits. Since, in a room of constant temperature, variations in skin temperature are a function of peripheral blood flow, information about the state of the vessels is transmitted to the organism on a moment-by-moment basis. The evidence is clear and mounting that, when placed in such a feedback loop, patients with Raynaud's syndrome can reliably learn to control voluntarily the dilation of these peripheral vessels.

However, it is not so clear that this model for the action of biofeedback will hold for activities predominantly innervated by the central nervous system. Certainly, this same argument can be made for neuromuscular reeducation work of various sorts. Indeed, one excellent way to describe the impact of biofeedback on Mr. T. is to say that the machine was used to place him in a negative biofeedback loop that retrained the relevant muscles of the head, neck and shoulders. (It is interesting to speculate on why these "voluntary" muscles cannot simply be relaxed without the aid of any equipment, since they are innervated by the central nervous system. Somehow the biofeedback seems to overcome the effects of habituation that make this task so difficult.)

But the same argument will not hold for many other health-related behaviors. For example, no one has yet provided convincing evidence that the application of biofeedback plays any particular role in correcting maladaptive eating, smoking, or drinking behavior. Of course, to the degree that these activities are stress-related and to the degree that biofeedback can be used in the management of such stress, a relationship can be established. However, that relationship is much more indirect and not nearly as impelling as the one that can be made for biofeedback-induced control of visceral activity. What I do wish to argue, however, is that the cybernetic model which underlies biofeedback also can be utilized to understand the principles under which these other health-related activities can be regulated.

Consider the change in the social roles of patient and doctor in health care when using biofeedback training as a model.

The most profound shift concerns the locus of responsibility for health care. In more traditional models, the physician is responsible for maintaining a healthy patient who is only responsible for following the physician's orders. In a health care model for which biofeedback training is the template, the responsibility for health care shifts to the patient. It becomes obvious when doing biofeedback training that the therapist does not, and cannot, control the dysregulated response. Rather, the patient develops an alternative mode of responding which provides mastery over the disorder. In the course of this development, it is the patient who, in a peculiar way, decides the course of the disorder by self-regulating what the body will do. For example, Mr. T. spoke once, toward the end of treatment, of being in a stressful situation and deciding that he was not going to get a headache because of it. The headache was successfully aborted.

It is inevitable that if the role of the patient changes, so must that of the clinician. In a health care system in which the goal is the training of patient self-regulation, questions may be asked about how the therapist functions. If biofeedback training is a model, two such functions emerge. The first is goal setting (education). One requirement for any self-regulated behavior is a clear specification of what is to be accomplished. Goals must be both relevant and reasonable and their specification may require technical information beyond the training of the patient. Mr. T., for example, having discovered the relation between myofacial chronic neck contraction and head pain, needed some instruction on the relation between chronic muscle contraction and habituation before he would accept the training paradigm.

The second function is to act as a trainer, or, if you will, facilitator for self-regulated behavior. The dimensions of such behavior remain to be determined in detail. However, some broad outlines seem to be clear, the most important of which is that such changes are simultaneously cognitive, emotional, and behavioral in character (Bandura, 1977).

It is only in recent years that the significance of cognitive factors in health has become clear (Mahoney, 1974). We have all had patients who explain continued smoking as being due to the fact that they believe they are too old to change. What has not been clear to such patients is the degree to which such beliefs provide the basis for resistance to good health care practices. The belief that one is not capable of changing one's behavior may be a strong factor in

preventing the behavior change from being initiated. Such beliefs
are often deeply rooted in the social, cultural, and psychological
history of the patient and are therefore strongly defended. However, as Michenbaum and his colleagues (1977) have shown, change in
belief structures is possible, with quite direct and predictable
changes in behavior. It is worth noting that such cognitive changes
may often be observed during biofeedback training. Patients who are
convinced of their inability to do anything about their arousal
levels sometimes change this belief as the electromyograph reports a
self-directed downward shift in muscle tension levels.

       Equally pervasive is the role of emotional factors in inducing
self-directed health care. Since the advent of work in psychosomatic medicine (see Alexander, 1950) there has been consensus among
investigators that emotional arousal can have consequences for the
well-being of a patient. Differences, of course, have existed concerning the theoretical treatment of this fact, but not about the
fact itself. What has not been treated well is the way in which
emotional arousal is translated into health care issues. Clearly,
emotional commitments can often stand in the way of behavior change.
An obese patient who is terrified at the prospect of going back into
the social swirl is less likely to manage a weight problem than one
who does not have that concern. Alternatively, a patient with high
self-esteem is far more likely to maintain positive health care
practices that one who is not. The problem for the patient is to
learn how to make deliberate effective changes in emotional state.
Again, biofeedback training can sometimes be useful, especially in
cases in which emotional expression has been somatically blocked.

       The role of behavior change itself in inducing positive health
care practices should also be considered. As a number of workers
have pointed out (see Bandura 1977(b)) behavior change itself can
produce predictable changes in emotional and cognitive processing,
which in turn produce further changes in behavior. For example,
post-myocardial infarction patients who exercise can often deal more
adequately with depression than those who do not. The induction of
such behavior change is a fascinating area of study, but its analysis is beyond the scope of this paper. It is clear that the initiation and maintenance of such changes are critical components of
self-regulated health care, and biofeedback training can be a powerful tool for initiating such behavior change (Pancheri et al.,
1979).

       I should like to close this paper with some comments directed
at the relation between biofeedback, self-regulated health care, and
medical practice. It has been argued that biofeedback represents an
example of a generalized control technique in nature, the negative
feedback loop. This technique, properly applied, should permit
patients to exercise greater control over their own health care.
The clinician in such a system functions as a facilitator in the

development of this self-control.

Decisions need to be made about when to employ biofeedback
training. The issue seems to me to be an empirical one, and concerns our understanding of the etiology of the disorder as well as
its immediate seriousness. Self-regulative strategies for health
care seem to be most useful in long-term stress reduction programs
and in those disorders in which stress plays an important etiological and perpetuating role.

DISCUSSION

PARTICIPANT: There was an article on migraine headaches. You
are probably familiar with it. In the conclusions here, about using
biofeedback as a mode of treatment, there is a statement —"however,
our second conclusion is that dramatic therapeutic improvement in
migraine headaches with hand temperature biofeedback is not due to a
specific property of skin temperature alterations, but rather is due
to nonspecific effects of clinical procedures employed. The
results of this double-blind study are negative not because the
treated group failed to improve, but because the two control groups
improved as much as the treated group did. Third, headache diary
keeping and attention from therapists and experimenters are likely
to be a part of these nonspecific effects." Would you comment on
this? Because the implication is that we don't need the machines.
We don't need anything else. All we need is a kind, sympathetic
clinician.

JACOBS: If migraine headache was totally curable by kind and
sympathetic clinicians, it wouldn't be so stubbornly resistant to
treatment. We're going to hear more about headaches before we're
done here. You'll probably get a headache from listening. My
understanding of biofeedback is that it really functions in two ways
which only partially overlap. One of those two ways is that it is
at times, and will be more so in the future, a tool directed at the
specific training of specific end organ systems for specific purposes. Period. That is the way it is used, for example, in neuromuscular reeducation where it's very clear what you are doing and
why you are doing it. And you're doing it because there isn't anything else that will do that for the end organ system. The second
use is somewhat more general. I think the problem that we get into
is that you don't need to do biofeedback to get that second effect.
At least not in all cases. That's that generalized kind of stress
reduction, that generalized kind of feeling better, the reduction of
the arousal state, the development, to use Stoyva's language, of a
cultivated state of low arousal which undoubtedly has an effect on a
number of different specific disorders. Now it is quite true that
in that second instance you don't need to use biofeedback. And
maybe for some patients, biofeedback is not the treatment of choice.

Right now that is a clinical matter. It is not clear why you ought to use biofeedback in some instances and not use it in others. I can only tell you that I read that paper. It's a good paper, by the way, and the people who did it are very competent people. I don't know how to square that conclusion away with the fact that I've had patients come into the office who have been treated by good, kind, competent clinicians who weren't using biofeedback, and whose headaches didn't go away. And we did precisely what was in the experiment as part of the experimental group and the headaches did go away. Now I don't think that that proves the universal efficacy of biofeedback. I think it says something about individual differences. And we don't have a fine-grained enough analysis yet to be able to discuss that in a meaningful way. But the paper is fascinating and I think we have to pay attention to it. It raises some serious issues for us.

PARTICIPANT: First let me preface this by saying that I come from the standpoint of being somewhat in support of biofeedback. In addressing the issue of total patient health care you talked a little bit about the nature of undefined issues and what causes disease. I'm wondering about the application of any specific agent, whether it's biofeedback, medicine, or surgery in the treatment of an illness without a more total program for the patient's health in terms of preventing future disease, which leads me basically to consider the question of symptom substitution.

JACOBS: I may have a blind spot somewhere in the way in which I see what happens to people I work with. I have never seen anybody get symptom substitution. That issue has been raised since biofeedback started. I have never seen it happen. It's conceivable that it could and maybe it happens and I don't see it. I have not seen it. The issue about setting up more general programs for patient care is a fascinating one. I don't know where the boundary conditions are for that kind of thing. I think you know that's kind of like saying you think that you like your mother sometimes or something. I mean, sure everybody would want to work to make sure that people don't get sick. That's a neat notion. The problem is to know what levels of intervention are effective, are cost effective, or time effective or relevant. I mean, if somebody comes in and he's got muscle contraction headaches, do you need to work on his bowel? I don't know. We can spend three sessions doing a very detailed analysis and that might be fun and it might even be helpful. I don't know. I do know that it's going to cost a lot of money and it's going to take a lot of time. I don't know where the balance is for that. And what I found is that when I do an intake, I find myself skimming over things and hoping to God I didn't miss something back there. That's a very real issue. I don't think that's a satisfactory answer, but it is the best I can give you at the moment. Thank you.

REFERENCES

Alexander, F. Psychosomatic medicine: Its principles and
    applications. New York: W.W. Norton & Co., 1950.
Bandura, A. Self-efficacy: Toward a unifying theory of behavioral
    change. Psychological Review, 1977(a), 84, 191-215.
Bandura, A. Social Learning theory. Englewood Cliffs, N.J.:
    Prentice-Hall, 1977(b).
Cannon, W. B. The wisdom of the body. New York: Norton, 1932.
Ellis, A. A rational-emotive approach to behavior change. In
    Burton, A. (Ed.), What makes behavior change possible? New
    York: Brunner/Mazel, 1976.
Mahoney, M. J. Cognition and behavior modification. Cambridge,
    Mass.: Balinger, 1974.
Meichenbaum, D. Cognitive behavior modification: An integrative
    approach. New York: Plenum, 1977.
Pancheri, P., Crebelli, M., & Chiari, G. Clinical application of
    EMG feedback in anxiety neurosis. In N. Birbaumer & H. D.
    Kimmel (Eds.), Biofeedback and self-regulation. Hillsdale,
    N.J.: Lawrence Erlbaum Associates, 1979.
Weiner, N. Cybernetics or control and communication in the animal
    and machine. Cambridge, Mass.: M.I.T. Press, 1948.

BEHAVIORAL APPLICATIONS IN THE ASSESSMENT OF HIGH BLOOD PRESSURE

Bernard T. Engel

Gerontology Research Center (Baltimore)
National Institute on Aging
National Institutes of Health, PHS
U.S. Department of Health and Human Services, Bethesda
Baltimore City Hospital
Baltimore, MD

High blood pressure is a clinical problem of epidemic proportions in Western societies (Julius & Schork, 1971). It is a physiological state which, if sustained, leads to vascular damage and
cardiomegaly. Among its eventual sequelae are such catastrophic
effects as renal parenchymal damage, cerebral vascular accidents or
myocardial infarctions. Furthermore, sustained high blood pressure
accelerates the development of atherosclerosis and the complications
of diabetes mellitus. Because a number of investigators have shown
that the autonomic nervous system plays a role in the expression of
the elevated pressure (Engel & Bickford, 1961; Frohlich, Tarazi, &
Dustan, 1969; Esler, Julius, Zweifler, Randall, Harburg, Gardiner, &
DeQuattro, 1977), a number of behavioral scientists and behaviorally
oriented clinicians have tried to bring their skills to bear on the
management of hypertensive patients. Some of the questions that
have been addressed include the role of social stressors in the
development (Gutman & Benson, 1971) or morbidity of hypertension
(Henry, Ely, Stephens, Ratcliffe, Santisteban, & Shapiro, 1971); the
role of behavioral management techniques in improving patient
adherence to medical advice (Haynes, Sackett, Gibson, Tayler,
Hackett, Robers, & Johnson, 1976); and the role of behavioral techniques in the control of blood pressure (Frumkin, Nathan, Prout, &
Cohen, 1978; Seer, 1979; Shapiro, Schwartz, Ferguson, Redmond, &
Weiss, 1977). Before one can undertake to investigate the role of
behavioral modification techniques in the control of hypertension,
he needs first to establish a reliable method for assessing blood
pressure. Clearly, before one can hope to measure the effectiveness
of an intervention, he first must define a set of outcome measures

on which to base his conclusions about therapeutic effectiveness, and he must then establish a baseline for these measures so that the effectiveness of his intervention can be assessed accurately. It will be the purpose of this paper to consider these two questions.

OUTCOME MEASURES

Two kinds of outcome measures have been extensively analyzed in the epidemiological literature: one is morbidity and the other is mortality (Kannel, 1974). Such epidemiological studies have been extremely valuable since they have shown how important it is to reduce blood pressure; however, these outcome measures are of limited value to a clinician since they are the outcomes he wishes to prevent. Clinical intervention in hypertension has focused pri- marily on strategies for reducing blood pressure, or in patients in whom morbid events already have occurred, on minimizing the progression of organ damage. Therefore, in this article I will limit my discussion to a consideration of blood pressure itself.

Blood pressure is difficult to assess because it is so variable. This fact has been documented in longitudinal studies carried out over many years (Engel & Malmstrom, 1967), in clinical studies carried out over many months (VA Cooperative Study Group, 1975) and in evaluative studies carried out over several weeks (Hypertension Cooperative Group, 1977). Findings such as these have caused investigators to focus on the definition of high blood pressure (Julius & Schork, 1971). For example, epidemiological studies have shown that blood pressure rises with age (Engel & Malmstrom, 1967; Julius & Schork, 1971) so that any arbitrary defi- nition of high blood pressure, e.g., 140/190 mm Hg., is likely to include age as an implicit correlate of blood pressure. Furthermore, because blood pressure is variable from occasion to occasion in the same person, it is possible to find that someone who is diagnosed as hypertensive on one visit will be judged normoten- sive on a second visit. At one time this so-called labile hyperten- sion was thought to be a precursor of fixed hypertension. However, it is now known that not all "labile hypertensives" develop fixed hypertension (Julius & Schork, 1971). This condition of lability often is called borderline hypertension, and it is recognized as a risk factor for hypertension, but it is neither a sufficient nor a necessary stage in the the natural history of the disorder.

There are several studies which indicate that blood pressure varies considerably through the day (Miller-Craig, Bishop, & Raftery, 1978; Littler, West, Honour, & Sleight, 1978), and varies also depending upon the circumstances of measurement (Hammarstrom, 1947). In particular, it has been reported that physicians obtain higher estimates of blood pressure than do non-physicians (Sokolow, Werdegar, Kain, & Hinman, 1966), and that blood pressure fluctuations throughout the day are correlated with self-ratings of mood (Sokolow, Werdegar, Perloff, Cowan, & Brenenstuhl, 1970; Whitehead, Blackwell, DeSilva, & Robinson, 1977). It also has been noted that when a patient records his own blood pressure, he often records values which are lower than those recorded by a physician (Ayman & Goldshine, 1940).

Taken together, all of these findings suggest that one should obtain estimates of blood pressure lability as well as blood pressure level; that these estimates should be made over an extended period to permit one to sample a range of circumstances and conditions; that these estimates should be taken throughout the day to allow for diurnal variations; and that blood pressure should be measured both by professional and nonprofessional observers. We have recently completed a study of 127 patients who monitored their blood pressures three times/day every day for about one month, and who also had their pressures recorded weekly by a professional (Engel, Gaarder, & Glasgow, 1981). In the next section I will review some of our findings.

BLOOD PRESSURE LEVELS

When patients are enrolled in a clinical study of blood pressure, it is a common finding that the pressures recorded during the study are lower than those recorded prior to the study, and that this is true even though no formal intervention has occurred (Hypertension Cooperative Group, 1977; Grenfell, Briggs, & Holland, 1963). In our study we found that not only were professionally measured blood pressure levels lower during the baseline month than they were before the baseline period, but also that the correlations between professional levels taken before and during the baseline period were quite low (systolic = .37; diastolic = .20). These data suggest strongly that there is a strong reactive component to professionally-determined blood pressure; that this reactive component habituates or extinguishes as a result of frequently repeated measurement; and that the degree of reactivity and/or habituation varies considerably among individuals, thus accounting for the small correlations cited above. Self-determined blood pressures vary systematically throughout the day. Both systolic and diastolic pressures are highest in the afternooon; however, systolic pressures rise from morning to evening whereas diastolic pressures fall over this same time period. In contrast to the professionally-determined pressures, the self-determined pressures are highly intercorrelated (systolic = .91; diastolic = .91) suggesting that these measures are highly reliable. In almost every patient, self-determined and professionally-determined blood pressure levels fall throughout the month. The degree of fall is correlated with the level of pressure: the higher the initial pressure, the greater the fall (systolic = .53; diastolic = .52). During the baseline month systolic pressure fell an

average of .3 mm Hg/day (9 mm Hg overall) and diastolic pressure
fell about .2 mm Hg/day (6 mm Hg overall).

BLOOD PRESSURE LABILITY

The concept of blood pressure lability is very confused in the
literature. Clinicians tend to think of lability as the differences
among pressure levels taken on several occasions, whereas scientists usually refer to a statistical index such as the standard
deviation to estimate lability. We looked at both of these indices,
and a third, the average daily range of systolic or diastolic pressure, as well. The results were quite interesting. Standard deviations of self-determined blood pressures were highly intercorrelated
(systolic = .76; diastolic = .73), and average daily blood pressure
range also correlated well with these measures (systolic = .62;
diastolic = .66). Changes in professionally recorded pressures were
not at all correlated with either the standard deviation of pressure
(systolic = .06; diastolic = -.02) or with average daily pressure
range (systolic = -.13; diastolic = .05). Thus, it would appear that
either the standard deviation of pressure or the daily range of
pressure would be a better index of lability than would be the
change in pressure level.

INDIVIDUAL DIFFERENCES

From a clinical point of view it is especially important to have
techniques which will enable one to assess a single patient. For
that reason I have selected the data for one patient for particular
study. This patient was a 28-year-old man whose prestudy, professionally measured blood pressure was 143/90 mm Hg. During the
baseline period his professionally-determined pressure during the
baseline period was 150/95. However, his self-determined pressures
were extremely variable throughout the day: in the morning his
pressure averaged 122/82; in the evening his pressure was 130/84;
and in the afternoon his pressure was 146/90. Clearly, this man
would have been judged normotensive during the morning and evenings,
but hypertensive both in the clinic and throughout most of the day.
Figure 1 shows his self-determined and professionally-determined
blood pressure levels during the entire baseline period. Note the
extent to which his self-determined, afternoon pressures and the
professionally-determined pressures differ from his self-determined,
morning, or evening pressure levels. In order to learn more about
the factors which might be mediating these blood pressure patterns,
I asked this man to measure his pressure once every hour, from the
time he awoke until noon for several weeks. Figure 2 shows the
results. During workdays his pressures rose consistently throughout
the morning to the hypertensive levels he typically measured during
the afternoons. However, on weekends or holidays, his average

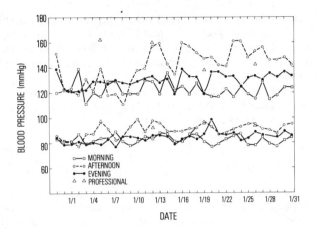

Figure 1

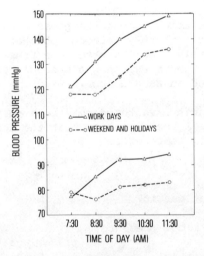

Figure 2

pressure levels were substantially lower: his noon readings were comparable to his average daily evening readings.

These data show strikingly that environmental factors can exercise clinically significant influences on blood pressure. However, it would never have been possible to learn that if we had not studied this patient systematically and thoroughly. It seems very clear to me that the strategy one would choose to treat a patient such as this would be vastly different if one collected data such as we did than if one relied merely on clinically measured blood pressure. Thus, the conclusions I wish to draw are that: 1) In order to understand behavior, we must take a thorough behavioral history and that is equally true whether the behavior is overt or physiological; 2) the method for obtaining behavioral data is the study of behavior, <u>in situ</u>; the clinic provides a very limited and biased environment in which to carry out such studies; and 3) at least in some patients, concurrent life events do exercise important influences on blood pressure.

DISCUSSION

PARTICIPANT: For several years I have been, on a clinical basis, having patients do baseline home recordings prior to either starting or changing any hypertensive medication and a lot of times I have difficulty in getting patients to get a three-time-a-day pressure for me. If you had to choose one or two determinations as being most indicative of round-the-clock main arterial pressure, which ones would you go for?

ENGEL: The correlations among the pressures throughout the day are extremely high so that they pattern together. If I were in that position, I would surely take the afternoon pressures because they'd be likely to be the highest and that's probably the sort of thing you're most interested in as a doctor.

PARTICIPANT: I just have three questions on your research data. First of all, I guess I heard you say that the modality you used for feedback was extremity temperature?

ENGEL: No.

PARTICIPANT: What was it?

ENGEL: Systolic blood pressure.

PARTICIPANT: And the larger drop on relaxation than the feedback. Was that when the feedback also was prior to the relaxation?

ENGEL: No, patients did one or the other for three months. Each time they did their thing, they measured their pressures before and then after. Each time, so for a single patient we may have 200 pre-post difference scores for a given patient in a three-month period. The change, from before to after relaxation, the change from before to after feedback, is what I am telling you about. On the average, in the course of, and I broke it up into monthly periods. O.K. Does that help you?

PARTICIPANT: I guess in the paradigm that I saw the people participated either first in a relaxation phase and then in a feedback phase or the other way around.

ENGEL: People participated. Let's take a hundred patients.
Twenty of them merely monitored their blood pressures for seven
months. They were the control group. Forty of them participated in
a relaxation phase for three months and forty of them participated
in a feedback phase for three months. At the end of that three
months half of each group crossed over and half of each group continued to do the same thing. So twenty of the patients who started
out relaxing actually relaxed for six months. Twenty of the
patients who started out relaxing went to feedback. O.K.?

PARTICIPANT: In the slide that showed the changes in the feedback period, which were also decreased changes, there seemed to be
greater variability. Was that so, did you see that during the
period of change while feedback was taking place? There was quite a
bit of variability in the blood pressure between sessions.

ENGEL: I've never looked at that. I can't answer that.

PARTICIPANT: Sir, in my office we use a blood pressure cuff
that is electronic: it beeps and with an electric flashing light
with each pulse. Have you had any experience with that?

ENGEL: When we set up to do this, we surveyed about a half
dozen electronic blood pressure devices and we found them
unreliable. So we rejected them all as being impractical in our
study. We went to this mechanical device which uses an anaroid
monometer and that's what we ended up with.

PARTICIPANT: Well, this one uses the anaroid monometer also,
but it gives a feedback of a flashing light and a beep at the same
time, so the patient, in using it in training, doesn't have to use a
stethoscope or learn how to hear those arterial sounds.

ENGEL: Well, again, our experience with those devices . . . we
tested several of them in the laboratory and we were dissatisfied
with their reliability in our hands and we thought to give these to
patients would probably result in chaos. They are also about twice
as expensive.

PARTICIPANT: That's true. One other question. I use a pulse
wave velocity machine, basically experimentally. Have you had any
experience with these, and in correlating blood pressure changes?

ENGEL: Well, I have not had experience, but I have looked at
this as a physiological phenomenon. I am not convinced that it is
going to be a valid measure of blood pressure because it depends on
what you mean when you talk about pulse wave velocity versus transit
time. If you mean pulse wave velocity measured between two points

in a vessel, then that's not a bad measure of pressure. If you mean the time from the R wave to the appearance of a pulse in the periphery, then that has a large component of the pre-ejection period in it. The pre-ejection period has nothing whatever to do with blood pressure. It's a measure of dP/dt. So I suspect that it will not prove to be a . . . It'll have a correlation like so many correlations in psychology are--.3.

PARTICIPANT: What is the commercial name of the instrument you use?

ENGEL: Yes, that is the Autosphyg made by Proper.

PARTICIPANT: The blood pressure you took nine times or they took nine times a day. How about the relaxation practice, was the frequency the same?

ENGEL: No, there was formal relaxation and informal relaxation. You remember I'd mentioned briefly that after six weeks into this, we asked the patients to try to do it briefly, in situ conditions? So we have no measure at all of how often they did that. None whatever. How many times the patient may have done that while sitting in a conference, while driving a car from one place to another, at a traffic light, all of those circumstances in which we urged the patient to try to do that - we have no data. We only have data on the formal practices when the patient actually took his blood pressure three times, then relaxed for anywhere from 30 seconds to 10 minutes, and then took his blood pressure again three times. Now, most patients . . . I guess, on the average there were large individual variations, but on the average I would say about three times every two days. At least once a day. The most common time of day to do it probably--I'm guessing now, but I think it's probably a good guess--would be the evening, with the afternoon being the time of day that we urged them to do it. I said to my patients, "Look we've done the baseline study. We now know when your pressure's highest. If you want to change your pressure, if this thing works which I don't know, but if it works, then it seems most sensible to try to use it at a time when the pressure is highest." So, I encouraged the patients to do it in the afternoon. Some patients did it three times a day; reported, that is. When I say they did it three times a day, what I mean is they took it three times before and three times after and sent us all those numbers every day. Some patients did it only once or twice a day. O.K.?

PARTICIPANT: I presume from what you've said that there were no specific conditions that a person was supposed to get in a certain state, or the professional was to help a certain person get in a certain state such as relaxing or running in place or whatever before the blood pressure was taken.

ENGEL: No. They might have been in their offices, if they were office workers or whatever they were doing.

PARTICIPANT: Given the data that you gave us, with differences between clinically measured blood pressure and self-determined blood pressure, I'm now wondering at what level I would begin to make interventions. You mentioned this a little bit, but have you done any bell shaped curves on a general population to determine what upper 10%, at what level you'll get that 10% cut-off or 5% cut-off or whatever?

ENGEL: I would be disinclined to do it on a statistical basis. I think that that in itself could take a lifetime. Because I would really be more interested in morbidity than mortality. I would be more interested in clinical outcome measures rather than statistical assessments. It's a whole new world.

PARTICIPANT: Do you have any correlation? You have your data there which suggests that perhaps 30-85 on a self-determined basis might correlate with 90-95 on a clinically determined basis.

ENGEL: The correlation between self-determined pressures and professionally determined pressures on the average is about 0.4 systolic, something like that, 0.4-0.5. So that's about 25% of the variance. It leaves a great deal to be desired. But the norms are on professionally measured pressures, not on self-determined pressures. But I think we need some self-determined norms, since they're measuring two different things. And certainly, anyone with experience with hypertensive patients is well aware that you see some patients in the office with high pressures and you get worried about them and twenty years later they're still coming in with high pressures and they don't look much different. At the same time, you'll see patients with relatively low pressures in the office who show a fulminating course. So it's clear while those data . . . while they are, if you've got nothing, that's better than nothing, are not completely adequate. And many doctors have turned to self-determination as a means of getting more information about the patient. But there are an awful lot of cheap experiments you can do. Like the example I gave of the patient who measured his pressures every half hour throughout the morning both during work days and nonwork days. That's a dramatic effect and it would suggest to me a different intervention strategy than if there were no difference.

PARTICIPANT: Could you say a little more about the biofeedback training per se - how many times did you encourage them to bring the blood pressure up and monitor it and then . . . ?

ENGEL: Well, typically they would take their three pressures for, let's say, the afternoon. Then they would pump the cuff up to

about systolic pressure, listen to the brachial artery sounds, and
try to make them go away over about a 25-second period. If the
brachial artery sounds could go away, then they would let the
pressure down, wait about 15 or 20 seconds. We warned them not to
maintain the cuff at near systolic pressure, then pump it back up.
Now try to make the brachial artery sounds go away. If they failed
on two consecutive trials, they were to give it up. If the pressure
. . . I warned everyone very carefully about that in the first
week. We didn't really care about the level of pressure. The
important thing was to develop the skill. So if the pressure went
up, that's not unreasonable. One would expect it to go up. Don't
worry about it. The important thing is to play with your blood
pressure. Incidentally, I also told patients in the baseline period
to play with their blood pressures. I have yet to see a hypertensive patient, and I've seen a lot of them, who doesn't have
notions about what makes the blood pressure go up and what makes the
blood pressure go down. I said, "This is your great chance to test
those notions. If you think a fight with your husband, in fact,
raises your blood pressure, go pick a fight, and then take your
blood pressure." (laughter)

PARTICIPANT: The other question I had was, did you fool around
with the other side of this? One can do it with diastolic pressure
bringing it down to a level where it has just disappeared and then
wait for the tone to come in.

ENGEL: I'm a little less confident about this and diastolic
pressure. I have never worked with it. A few people have and it's
in the literature. And I don't have any data that say it shouldn't
be done, but my experience is that it is a lot harder to take
diastolic pressure. In a significant number of people it just fades
away like old soldiers but it never dies. And in some people you
get a very potent muffling effect, but you don't get a good
disappearance. We tried to use phase five disappearance, but I find
it less reliable than systolic. Systolic is very sharp. There is
nothing, and then there's something and you can get very good
agreement. Now remember we never brought a patient into the
laboratory. The whole training was done within a one-hour office
visit. We tried to make this both a research project and practical
program at the same time. I can teach most anyone, I think, to
recognize systolic pressure if he's not deaf. But diastolic would
be very difficult in this feedback mode. I think it would be. At
least more difficult.

PARTICIPANT: I have a question. What was the age range of the
patients you studied in this particular group?

ENGEL: 28-73.

PARTICIPANT: O.K. That's interesting because in my own clinical practice I find that the lability, in some ways, is related to age. And that I wonder, in patients who have had documented hypertension for 10 or more years, how much of an effect you can achieve by this method?

ENGEL: Let me talk a little bit about that. I didn't present the age data from the baseline period. With respect to systolic pressure there is a correlation between blood pressure level, between standard deviation, between range of blood pressure, and age for systolic pressure. There is no relationship in diastolic pressure. So there is a consistent relationship between systolic pressure indices. Whether level or lability and age there is no relationship in our experience between diastolic pressure and lability. Ah, the correlation between prebaseline and baseline professional difference and age is negative, that is to say the largest difference between prebaseline and baseline professionally measured pressures occurs in the younger people. So what I think you're seeing, is a habituation in the . . . we also see that the slope, the fall in blood pressure throughout the baseline period, is correlated with age. The older people having the greater fall and that's also correlated with pressure level. The higher you start the greater your fall. All right? So what I'm trying to say is that there are two processes operating. There is a habituation of blood pressure as a result of frequent measurement and that habituation is correlated with age. The older people, in general, show more habituation than younger people. At the same time, there's an iatrogenic response to the taking of blood pressure that's negatively correlated with age. Young people show a greater reactivity to professionally measured blood pressure than do older people. So you have to extinguish, if you want to talk about a study, the iatrogenic reaction, the iatrogenically induced, elicited response and at the same time permit the blood pressure to habituate as a result of frequent self-determination. Both these processes are operating at the same time, I think.

PARTICIPANT: The second part of my question is, did any of these patients get followed for a lengthy period of time and is this a practical modality? Do these people have to have weekly or monthly sessions with you or an individual like you in order to maintain the beneficial effects of blood pressure lowering?

ENGEL: Well, this was an experiment.

PARTICIPANT: But has it been pursued?

ENGEL: Well, it's in the process of being done. Most patients we saw three times in each phase: at the beginning of each phase, in the middle of the phase, and the end of the phase. Occasionally we saw patients more often than that usually to exchange a blood pressure cuff which was damaged or not working or sometimes because

the patient, very rarely, the patient wasn't managing the skills.
We could see the data coming in and they were bizarre. So we would
schedule another meeting. In general, the patient was seen at the
beginning, six weeks, and one month. In that sense, in a HMO
setting with health associates or other professional, paramedical (I
don't like that word, but anyway) professionals, I think it's practical to do that. Does that answer your question?

Subsequent to this presentation, we have reported on the treatment phase of our study (Glasgow, M. S., Engel, B. T., & Gaarder,
K. R. Behavioral treatment of high blood pressure: II. Acute and
sustained effects of relaxation and systolic blood pressure biofeedback. Psychosomatic Medicine, in press)

The following is the abstract from that report:

The effects on blood pressure of regular patient and professional monitoring of blood pressure, extensive patient-involved
assessment of results, relaxation, and systolic blood pressure biofeedback are analyzed by comparisons of data from two three-month
treatment periods with results from a one-month baseline period and
by comparisons among control and treatment groups. Ninety borderline hypertensive patients completed the treatments. Major findings
are: A. Acute effects; 1) Both relaxation and systolic blood
pressure biofeedback lowered blood pressure acutely. 2) Improvement
in performance of relaxation and biofeedback with practice showed
that they are learned skills. 3) Acutely, relaxation and biofeedback were equally effective for lowering systolic blood pressure,
but relaxation lowered diastolic blood pressure more. B. Long-term
effects; 1) Blood pressure declined for at least six months with
regular monitoring and patient-involved assessment. 2) The greatest
lowering of blood pressure by behavioral intervention occurred
during periods when pressures tended to be highest. 3) A combination of relaxation and biofeedback, with biofeedback preceding
relaxation, was better than either used alone and slightly, but not
significantly, better than relaxation preceding biofeedback. 4) The
long-term effects of biofeedback were slightly greater than those of
relaxation. A staged, incremental behavioral treatment of borderline hypertension is proposed.

REFERENCES

Ayman, D., & Goldshine, A. D. Blood pressure determinations
        by patients with essential hypertension. I. The dif-
        ference between clinic and home reading before
        treatment. American Journal of Medical Science, 1940,
        200, 465-474.

Engel, B. T., & Bickford, A. F. Stimulus-response and
     individual-response specificity in essential
     hypertensives. Archives of General Psychiatry, 1961, 5,
     478-489.
Engel, B. T., Gaarder, K. R., & Glasgow, M. S. Behavioral
     treatment of high blood pressure: I. Intra- and inter-
     daily variations of blood pressure during a one-month,
     baseline period. Psychosomatic Medicine, in press.
Engel, B. T., & Malmstrom, E. J. An analysis of blood pressure
     trends based on annual observations of the same
     subjects. Journal of Chronic Diseases, 1967, 20, 29-43.
Esler, M., Julius, S., Zweifler, A., Randall, O., Harburg, E.,
     Gardiner, H., & DeQuattro, V. Mild high-renin essential
     hypertension: Neurogenic human hypertension? New
     England Journal of Medicine, 1977, 296, 405-411.
Frohlich, E. D., Tarazi, R. C., & Dustan, H. P. Hyperdynamic
     B-adrenergic circulatory state. Archives of Internal
     Medicine, 1969, 123, 1-7.
Frumkin, K., Nathan, R. J., Prout, M. F., & Cohen, M. C.
     Nonpharmacologic control of essential hypertension in
     man: A critical review of the experimental literature.
     Psychosomatic Medicine, 1978, 40, 294-320.
Grenfell, R. F., Briggs, A. H., & Holland, W. C. Antihyper-
     tensive drugs evaluated in a controlled double-blind
     study. Southern Medical Journal, 1963, 56, 1410-1416.
Gutmann, M. C., & Benson, H. Interaction-of environmental fac-
     tors and systemic arterial blood pressure: A review.
     Medicine, 1971, 50, 543-553.
Hammarstrom, S. Arterial hypertension. I. Variability of
     blood pressure; II. Neurosurgical treatment, indications
     and results. Acta Medica Scandinavica (Suppl. 192) 1947,
     301 pp.
Haynes, R. B., Sackett, O. L., Gibson, E. S., Tayler, D. W.,
     Hackett, B. C., Robers, R. S., & Johnson, A. L.
     Improvement of medication compliance in uncontrolled
     hypertensives. Lancet, 1976, 1, 1265-1268.
Henry, J. P., Ely, D. L., Stephens, P. M., Ratcliffe, H. L.,
     Santisteban, G. A., & Shapiro, A. P. The role of psycho-
     social factors in the development of arteriosclerosis in
     DBA mice. Atherosclerosis, 1971, 14, 203-218.
Hypertension Detection and Follow-up Program Cooperative Group.
     Blood pressure studies in 14 communities. A two-stage
     screen for hypertension. Journal of the American Medical
     Association, 1977, 237, 2385-2391.
Julius, S., & Schork, M. A. Borderline hypertension--A critical
     review. Journal of Chronic Diseases, 1971, 23, 723-754.
Kannel, W. B. Role of blood pressure in cardiovascular mor-
     bidity and mortality. Progress in Cardiovascular
     Diseases, 1974, 17 (No.1), 5-24.

Littler, W. A., West, M. J., Honour, A. J., & Sleight, P.   The
        variability of arterial pressure. American Heart
        Journal, 1978, 95, 180–186.
Miller-Craig, M. W., Bishop, C. N., & Raftery, F. B.
        Circadian variation of blood pressure. Lancet, 1978,
        April, 795–797.
Seer, P.   Psychological control of essential hypertension:
        Review of the literature and methodological critique.
        Psychological Bulletin, 1979, 86, 1015–1043.
Shapiro, A. P., Schwartz, G. E., Ferguson, D. C. E., Redmond,
        D.P., & Weiss, S. M.   Behavioral methods in the treatment
        of hypertension. A review of their clinical status.
        Annals of Internal Medicine, 1977, 86, 626–636.
Sokolow, M., Werdegar, D., Kain, H. K., & Hinman, A. T.
        Relationship between level of blood pressure measured
        casually and by portable recorders and severity of
        complications in essential hypertension.   Circulation,
        1966, 34, 279–298.
Sokolow, M., Werdegar, D., Perloff, D. B., Cowan, R. M., &
        Brenenstuhl, H.   Preliminary studies relating portably
        recorded blood pressures to daily life events in
        patients with essential hypertension.   In M. Koster, H.
        Musph, & P. Visser (Eds.), Psychosomatics in essential
        hypertension.   Basel, Munchen, New York: Karger, 1970,
        pp. 1–189.
Veterans Administration Cooperative Study Group on Antihyper-
        tensive Agents.   Return of elevated blood pressure after
        withdrawal of antihypertensive drugs.   Circulation,
        1975, 51, 1107–1113.
Whitehead, W. E., Blackwell, B., DeSilva, H., & Robinson, A.
        Anxiety and anger in hypertension. Journal of
        Psychosomatic Research, 1977, 21, 383–389.

BIOFEEDBACK IN PULMONARY REHABILITATION

Brian L. Tiep

Director of Pulmonary Rehabilitation
City of Hope Medical Center
Duarte, California

Respiratory biofeedback resides in the domain of pulmonary rehabilitation. A true understanding of respiratory specific biofeedback must include an understanding of the environment for that therapy. Respiratory biofeedback is not a solitary form of therapy; rather it is a part of a large multimodal team approach to pulmonary rehabilitation. The greater goal is to improve the patients' ability to adapt to their illnesses by optimizing mental and physical functioning consistent with their pulmonary impairment. Pulmonary rehabilitation treats chronic obstructive lung diseases such as emphysema, chronic bronchitis, and bronchial asthma. The rehabilitation approach is based on the fact that in these chronic conditions the patients adapt by becoming increasingly sedentary, dependent upon others, and reconciled to progressive deterioration. Somewhere in the course of their disease, they enter a vicious cycle of impairment causing disability, causing slowing down, causing more disability. One cannot, therefore, simply treat the physical or the mental portion of this process in exclusion of the other. For therapy to be effective, patients require a thorough comprehension of their disease, the limits of their functional capacity, proper diet, medication, smoking, exercise for both endurance and strength building, and biofeedback techniques. Endurance exercise is a key to improving physical functioning.

Only a part of the patient's progressive inactivity and uninvolvement can be attributed to disease, for, as impaired as their lungs become, their cardiovascular conditioning is often worse. That is to say, the patient is actually limited by poor cardiovascular fitness. Thus, the pulmonary rehabilitation team has an excellent opportunity to improve the patient's ability to function by concentrating on cardiovascular conditioning.

Emphysema is often complicated by bronchopulmonary infection, mucous plugs, cor pulmonale (cardiac problems as a result of chronic lung disease), and congestive heart failure (as a result of cor pulmonale). These complications are major factors in the symptoms suffered by our patients. The usual medical approach is to stabilize these complications prior to subjecting the patient to rehabilitative care. However, there are several advantages to overlapping rehabilitation and acute medical care. First, patients can more effectively learn to recognize early signs and symptoms of their developing complications, which affords them the opportunity to seek help prior to deterioration. Second, patients beginning the program at their lowest functional level will be able to appreciate greater improvement in a shorter period of time. This improves patient motivation and self-concept. Third, the rehabilitation team becomes more realistically involved in the complex psychological presentation of these patients. The best rehabilitation management requires an intense, highly structured, continuous therapy aimed at realistically altering the patient's life style. In our hospital, the program is an in-patient program. There are a number of pulmonary rehabilitation practitioners who strongly support an outpatient approach, their most compelling argument being economic. In our experience, to maximize our rehabilitative results, the program structure requires 24 hour support for about three weeks. In such a high intensity program, patients get into difficulty most often at night. It is important and sometimes critical that there are trained personnel present during these difficult times. Our experience also shows that three weeks is the usual time span required for rehabilitation of patients with emphysema. Our patients often make rapid improvement during the first week of the program as they begin to recognize and appreciate their prior capability to function. However, during the second week, they are tired and sore from the first week. They might feel worse than they did when they started the program. They become rebellious, hostile, passive-aggressive, and tend to sabotage their management by becoming resistive to the program. We refer to this as the "second week syndrome." Patients are appropriately monitored and encouraged to pursue. Making it to the third week, they again show rapid progress and more fully appreciate their accomplishments both physically and emotionally.

The pulmonary rehabilitation team at the City of Hope Medical Center includes the physician, pulmonary rehabilitation nurse, psychologist consultant, and the patient. Each member of the team is a specialist and is considered a full colleague of the physician. Each team member conducts classes and individual sessions with the patient, and all major patient care decisions are team decisions. The team coordinator is a registered nurse who specializes in pulmonary rehabilitation.

Patients with chronic obstructive pulmonary disease are referred by their private physicians for pulmonary rehabilitation.

They undergo complete evaluation by the physician as well as other members of the team. Based on the team's physiological and psycho-social screening studies, they are accepted into the program. Patients sign a "contract" binding them to all aspects of the program. A breach of this contract results in early discharge from the program. A reasonable set of goals is prepared by the patient and the team, which becomes the basis for all further care. We often involve the patient's family in our teaching program so that both the patient and family learn techniques for coping outside the hospital.

Patients improve their physical functioning by endurance training. They are initially evaluated using a bicycle ergometer stress test sufficient to challenge their cardio-pulmonary system. The ergometer resistance is increased minute by minute while the physician monitors the patient's cardiogram. From this incremental test we are able to ascertain the safety of subjecting patients to exercise. While most endurance exercise improves the patient's cardiovascular fitness if done properly, the benefits of each exercise tends to be specific in both strength and endurance. Therefore, patients are subjected to both upper and lower extremity endurance training. The lower extremity training consists of walking, with increases of the patient's continuous walking time; the goal is to improve both endurance and pacing. It is not unusual for a patient to enter the program unable to walk for more than five minutes continuously (at any pace) and after three weeks rehabilitation, walk for 45 to 60 minutes. The upper extremity training uses an arm bicycle in which the patient's work load can be set. The total work is measured as watt minutes, which is the work load in watts multiplied by the number of minutes of continuous effort. The mechanisms for improvement are increased motivation, desensitization to dyspnea, improved mechanical efficiency, improved endurance of limb muscles, and improved endurance of ventilatory muscles.

Patients undergo a nutritional status evaluation complete with anthropomorphic measurement, serum proteins, and blood counts. Not all emphysema patients are underweight; in fact, some are rather obese. In either case, these patients are malnourished. Many patients have specific nutritional needs. All patients become actively involved in their dietary planning, hopefully leading to good nutrition at home.

Of course, no patient is allowed to smoke, since this is most often the cause of the illness in the first place. Therefore, all our patients are non-smokers when they enter the hospital.

Eighty to ninety percent of our patients do well in the hospital; however, when they leave the hospital and re-enter the real world, they understandably turn their attention to other pursuits. Transference of knowledge and skills acquired in the hospital to the

home setting becomes a critical issue. Thus, we have outpatient
follow-up which attends to the problem of continued compliance. It
includes physical therapy, occupational therapy, and regular clinic
visits with the nurse coordinator and physician along with other
pertinent team members utilizing graphing techniques to pinpoint
progress and provide encouragement.

The pulmonary rehabilitation program described in the foregoing
is the total therapeutic management for patients with obstructive
lung disease. It is multimodal and one of the modes is respiratory
biofeedback. The goal of biofeedback is to help patients understand
and modify their physiological function towards optimization. The
understanding and design of biofeedback systems for these patients
requires some understanding of the physiology. One should note that
all of our discussion will be directed toward biofeedback aimed at
modifying specific respiratory physiology. The most common usage of
the term biofeedback would almost make it synonymous with general
body relaxation. While we believe that relaxation can be helpful to
our patients, we feel that the most rewarding approach is to teach
the patient to modify the specific physiology of the respiratory
tract. All of our biofeedback monitoring is noninvasive, so we avoid
using monitoring techniques which modify the function they are monitoring. We will first take a look at the respiratory tract, its
anatomy, physiology, and pathology as they relate to biofeedback.

The lung resides in the chest cage and is housed in a sac known
as the pleural sac. There is a branching tree of tubing which com-
municates the air exchange areas of the lung with the outside
atmosphere via the naso-oropharynx. Through the naso-oropharnx,
atmospheric gases are drawn into the trachea, which bifurcates into
the right and left bronchi, supplying the right and left lung
respectively. These major bronchi in turn bifurcate many times
(similar to the branching of a tree), ending in the terminal bron-
chioles and finally into clusters of interconnecting alveoli. There
are some 750 million alveoli in the lungs of persons free of respiratory disease. Each alveolus is surrounded by a network of
capillaries through which air exchange between the air sacs and the
circulatory system takes place. The task of the lung is to exchange
oxygen and carbon dioxide with the blood stream, while the job of
the cardiovascular system is to distribute oxygen to all portions of
the body. While in the neighborhood of the bodily tissues, carbon
dioxide, an end product of metabolism, is gathered and conveyed via
the blood stream to the alveoli and thus returned to the atmosphere.

Any factor which impedes oxygen-carbon dioxide transport presents a problem, not only with oxygenation of all the tissues but
also in the delicate acid-base balance of the bloodstream and the
body in general. While there are many maladies which can impair
this delicate system, we shall turn our attention to air flow
obstruction in the bronchial passages.

We can characterize air flow obstruction in two ways: 1) dynamic obstruction, and 2) passive airways collapse. Dynamic obstruction occurs when the bronchial passages are actively constricted. These passages are tethered by smooth muscle. The effect of contracting these muscles is to grip and constrict the airways, thus causing obstruction to air flow. This situation is known as bronchospasm and is a major feature of bronchial asthma. Essentially, bronchospasm may be described as "twitchy" bronchial muscles and there are many possible triggering mechanisms for episodic bronchospasm. Examples of such triggers are: cigarette smoke, cold air, dust particles, allergens, infection, running, and emotional frustration.

The autonomic nervous system plays an important role in the regulation of bronchial motor tone. The studies of Spector and Luparello (McFadden, Luparello, Lyons, & Bleecker, 1969; Spector, Luparello, Kopetzky, Souhrada, & Kinsman, 1976) have demonstrated the influence of suggestion on both the stimulation and reversal of bronchospasm. From these studies we can conclude that higher centers in the brain are capable of modifying bronchomotor tone in either direction. It is reasonable to use a biofeedback training control approach to bronchospasm, since the bronchial passages are supplied by cholinergic fibers from the vagus nerve (Nadel, 1976). Vagal efferent innervation has been demonstrated to modify bronchomotor tone, and this effect can be blocked by such agents as atropine. Vachon and Feldman (Vachon & Rich, 1976; Feldman, 1976) taught their patients to reduce airway resistance by means of a computer assisted biofeedback signal which measures lung resistance by forced oscillation techniques. We have designed a biofeedback monitor which is sensitive to breath sound amplitude and produces a tone the frequency of which is proportional to the breath sound amplitude (Tiep, Alaniz, & Cordell, 1976). It consists of a contact microphone which is positioned over the trachea and senses breath sounds (Figure 1). This signal is passed through an averaging network which produces a voltage proportional to breath sound amplitude. A voltage to frequency converter produces the aforementioned tone. A visual display via a volt meter corresponds to the tone. This instrument is also capable of presenting amplified breath sounds to the patient. The value of this latter feature is to help the patient relate the biofeedback training to the specific physiological event. Bronchial asthma is episodic, that is to say, at one moment the patient may be completely free of symptoms and at the very next moment there might be an acute exacerbation. In order for patients to learn control over their asthma, we induce bronchospasm by treadmill exercise, which they will learn to control. The treadmill speed is adjusted so as to raise the cardiac frequency to 75 to 80% of maximum predicted heart rate. The patient wears a nose clip during the exercise in order to insure mouth breathing, thus potentiating the bronchoconstrictor effect to the exercise. After the exercise, the patient rests for 5 to 6 minutes, during which time

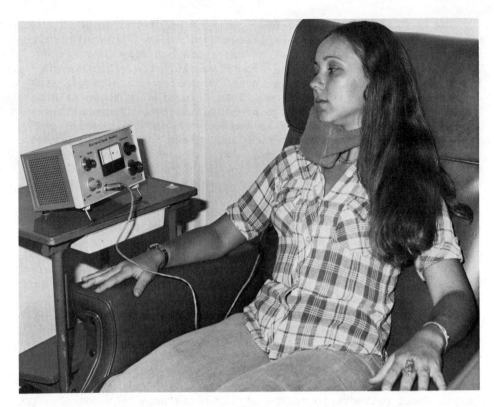

Figure 1

exercise induced asthma becomes manifest. He is then tested with
pulmonary function tests after which he receives biofeedback
training. After the training session, we repeat the pulmonary function tests. This biofeedback training requires 6 to 12 training
sessions to achieve full benefit. We have done studies which
demonstrated the relationship between breath sound amplitude and
airway obstruction. Of course, it is possible to have bronchospasm
of such severity as to cause extreme limitation in air flow, thereby
actually reducing breath sound amplitude. At this extreme, the
patient is severely compromised and requires more than a biofeedback
training session. In a recent study (manuscript in preparation), we
demonstrated that breath sound biofeedback was as effective as
inhaled aerosolized isoproterenol, and both were better than relaxation and suggestion in reversing bronchospasm. Using biofeedback,
the improvement in bronchospasm was 30% as measured by the forced
expiratory volume in one second (FEV_1); however, there was only a
15% improvement using suggestion. The biofeedback subjects improved
to their pre-exercise level following biofeedback training.

The other major cause of airway obstruction is passive collap-
sibility. The tendency for collapse of the smaller airway during
exhalation occurs due to the loss of elastic support tissues in
patients with pulmonary emphysema. In normal lungs, the higher
alveolar pressures maintain the smaller airways open during exhalation because of elastic recoil.   In the emphysema patient this
elastic recoil is reduced, so the smaller airways tend to collapse.
This tendency for airways to collapse is more pronounced when the
expiratory effort is impulsive. In addition, once the airways
collapse, further increase in positive intrapleural pressure results
in continued collapse, partly due to the venturi effect of rapid
flow (though the volume is small) through the small orifices. It
has been long accepted and taught in pulmonary rehabilitation programs that judicious use of back pressure techniques such as pursed-
lip breathing during the expiratory phase appear to help keep the
airway from collapsing. Many patients learn this method on their
own and they are probably more proficient at avoiding airway collapse than those who have to be instructed in it. The reason for
this is that those patients have learned to feel the delicate
balance between driving pressure and back pressure. In teaching
this method to emphysema patients, it is difficult if not impossible
to tell the patients exactly how much back pressure and driving
pressure to use. We have therefore designed a biofeedback technique
specifically aimed at teaching patients to minimize the variation in
intrathoracic pressure in the hope that they can learn that delicate
balance, thus reducing their work and energy cost of breathing.

Let us look at the work of breathing:

$$\text{Work of Breathing} \quad \text{W.O.B.} = \int_{0}^{V} P dV$$

where P = Pressure
V = Volume

For similar volumes, a reduction in intrathoracic pressure would be
expected to reduce the work and therefore the energy cost of
breathing. We have described a method of looking at intrathoracic
pressure non-invasively by a device which measures pressure-
displacement on the suprasternum. It consists of a plunger-sensor
supported by a recoil spring which floats in a plastic ring. The
plastic ring is attached by an adjustable arm to a stable platform
which is taped securely to the firm sternal portion of the chest
wall. The output of this device can be read as either total
pressure displacement or singly as the inspiratory or expiratory
pressure displacement. The visual output is a voltage reading and
the audio output is a variable frequency tone (Figure 2). In some
early studies, we demonstrated a linear relationship with pressure
as measured by a balloon in the esophagus connected to a pressure
transducer (Tiep, Mittman, & Trippe, 1977). The pressure displacement readings can be calibrated as alveolar pressure by equilibra-

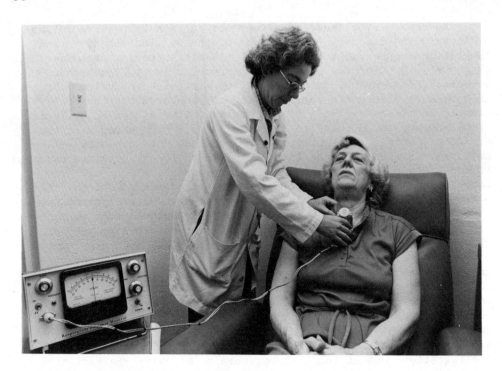

Figure 2

ting it against mouth pressure while the patient breathes against a
closed shutter with an open epiglottis. Our studies demonstrated a
24% mean reduction in suprasternal pressure displacement accompanied
by clinical improvement in these patients' abilities to control
their breathing patterns. Further clinical investigation in this
area is planned.

    In conclusion, biofeedback is a training approach in which spe-
cialized instruments are used to inform and continually update
patients about their physiological functions in such a manner that
they can modify those functions. It is an inner-body skill analogous to typing or riding a bicycle--both examples of somatically
controlled function. Neurophysiologists dub the nervous system that
controls these inner functions "autonomic," inferring automatic.
Since the early days of biofeedback, we have now come to accept that
instrumental control over vaso-motor responses, heart rate, blood
pressure, and a host of other physiological functions is possible
both in the research lab and in the clinical situation. Basmajian
demonstrated that it was possible to effect control in training of
single motor units and individual nerve cells (Basmajian, 1963a,
1963b). From his data and from the early studies on blood pressure
and heart rate, we now conclude that biofeedback can be a rather

specific technique. It is not always a potent technique. The ability to learn self-control over physiological functions depends upon
many factors, some of which are not yet understood. The motivation
of the patient coupled with the concern and technical skill of the
therapist help to determine the possible success or failure of such
self-control techniques.

DISCUSSION

PARTICIPANT: One of the problems of the emphysema patient is
that he often seems to have a reduced tidal volume. What would you
say about the probability of outcome if one were to take such
patients and teach them merely to breathe more slowly? Would that
have a probability, because of the requirement of the fixed amount
of air, to show increased tidal volume as a result of that type of
biofeedback that might be tried?

TIEP: In the very severe emphysema patient, tidal volume
reduction could be a problem. In the not so severe emphysema
patient that is not so much the problem; rather, it's the amount of
effort-pressure required to move that same volume. But in any case,
you're right that a reduction in respiratory rate is helpful. But
it shouldn't be only the reduction in respiratory rate, it should be
how that person breathes. People can develop back pressure techniques. They are taught this in rehabilitation programs. They're
taught pursed-lip breathing. This is where you breathe in through
your nose or your mouth, and then breathe out against pursed lips.
What you do is you provide a back pressure and that back pressure
tends to keep the airways open. We strongly suspect that patients
on this type of biofeedback are maximizing back pressure techniques.
In any case, it needs to be a smooth respiratory cycle. If they
breathe impulsively, then they are going to clamp down those airways
and when they do that they tend to follow through with very forceful
breathing. And when they do that, they make matters worse.

PARTICIPANT: Following up from that, might it be possible to
provide feedback by just simply monitoring chest or abdominal girth
and then having the individual try to produce smoother respiratory
cycles without the kind of forced breathing that you showed, by using
a visual or auditory indicant of the nature of the respiratory cycle
itself?

TIEP: Yes. In fact, that was the direction that I was going
in before I came up with the work of breathing biofeedback technique. I was really looking for kind of the bottom line indication
of whether the person was increasing or decreasing his intrathoracic
pressure for the same volume. That's a very reasonable approach and
we'll probably investigate it.

PARTICIPANT: Yes, I was wondering if you ever teach the

patients how to use a stethoscope as a way of monitoring their raw
respiratory signs as a feedback system.

TIEP: Yes, we do. What we do is we teach them on the biofeedback device and then we follow through with the use of the stethoscope. There is something else you can do though. If everybody
would put your fingers in your ears, in other words, occlude the
external sounds, the external environment, you can hear yourselves
breathing. Even over my talking, you can each hear yourself
breathing. And you can use your own fingers as part of a biofeedback system.

PARTICIPANT: I was wondering about how many treatment sessions
were necessary before you felt an individual actually gained control
and could alter his respiratory response to stress? And also, do
you ever combine relaxation training with biofeedback and what
results do you have?

TIEP: We found that eight treatment sessions was a very good
number and they should probably be done consecutively--maybe
skipping a weekend. With respect to relaxation, no we haven't. And
I'm constantly asked that question: whether we're really doing any
relaxation training. We're not using biofeedback as relaxation
training. We do have an occupational therapist who has specialized
in a progressive relaxation technique, and that has been helpful to
a number of our patients, but we're not giving it as part of the
biofeedback training. Our gut level feeling is that we don't think
it's really necessary. If a person can learn how to control asthma
attacks, he develops a certain amount of confidence, providing that
he really wanted to get rid of these asthma attacks. There are some
patients who thought that they did, but after a while they recognized that the asthma itself was kind of a friend to them and they
really missed that friend. They grieved over that friend. This is
not the majority of patients, however. But we've had some really
startling cases like that.

REFERENCES

Basmajian, J. V. Conscious control of single nerve cells.
       New Scientist, 1963, 20, 662-664. (a)
Basmajian, J. V. Control and training of individual motor
       units. Science, 1963, 141, 440-441. (b)
Feldman, G. M. The effect of biofeedback training on
       respiratory resistance of asthmatic children.
       Psychosomatic Medicine, 1976, 38 (1).
McFadden, Jr., E. R., Luparello T., Lyons H. A., & Bleecker, E.
       The mechanism of action of suggestion in the induction
       of acute asthma attacks. Psychosomatic Medicine, 1969,
       31, 134-143.

Nadel, J. A. Airways: Autonomic regulation and airway
    responsiveness. In Bronchial Asthma. Mechanisms and
    Therapeutics. Boston: Little Brown & Company. 1976,
    155-161.

Spector, S., Luparello, T. J., Kopetzky, M. T., Souhrada, J., &
    Kinsman, R. A. Response of asthmatics to methacholine
    and suggestion. American Review of Respiratory Disease,
    1976, 12, 43-49.
Tiep, B. L., Alaniz, J., & Cordell, J. Respiratory Feedback:
    Two non-invasive approaches in the treatment of patients
    with chronic obstructive disease. Proceedings of the
    San Diego Biomedical Symposium, 1976, 15, 371-374.
Tiep, B. L., Mittman, C., & Trippe, M. A new biofeedback
    technique for controlling intrathoracic pressure in
    patients with pulmonary emphysema. Proceedings of the
    San Diego Biomedical Symposium, 1977, 16, 215-220.
Vachon, L., & Rich, E. S. Visceral learning in asthma.
    Psychosomatic Medicine, 1976, 38 (2), 122-130.

PATHOGENESIS OF VASCULAR HEADACHES

Lee Kudrow

Director, California Medical Clinic for Headache
Encino, California

To the clinician treating primary headache disorders, appreciation of pathophysiologic mechanisms is not less important than
his recognition of diagnostic characteristics. Indeed, both aspects
are prerequisites to successful management of chronic or recurrent
headache patients. Thus, although the major thrust of this presentation concerns the mechanisms of vascular headaches, a clinical
review of all primary headache disorders is included.

CLASSIFICATION AND CLINICAL DESCRIPTIONS (TABLES 1 AND 2)

Migraine

Migraine affects women at least twice as often as men (Waters &
O'Connor, 1975). A positive family history of headache is found in
60-80% of patients (Goodell, Lewontin, & Wolf, 1954). Generally,
the age of onset is between late teens and early twenties. Attacks
occur with a frequency of one to three times a month, each lasting
as short as six to eight hours or as long as three days. The pain
is moderately severe, often throbbing, unilateral in 80% of cases;
and associated with nausea, vomiting, photophobia, and sonophobia.
Prodromes are characteristically described as scintillating scoto-
mata of 20-30 minutes duration, and when present, classify migraine
as the classical type.

Cluster Headache

The mean age at onset of cluster headache is 29 years. It
affects males five times as often as females (Kudrow, 1980).

In episodic cluster headache, attacks occur one to several
times a day for a six to twelve week period, followed by a

41

Table 1

```
MIGRAINE
    CLASSICAL
    COMMON
    OPHTHALMIC
    OPHTHALMOPLEGIC
    HEMIPLEGIC
    BASILAR ARTERY
    EQUIVALENTS ?

CLUSTER
    EPISODIC
    CHRONIC
        PRIMARY
        SECONDARY
        CPH
    ATYPICAL VARIANTS

SCALP MUSCLE CONTRACTION
    ACUTE
    CHRONIC

COMBINATION

POST-TRAUMATIC
    TYPES 1-4

CONVERSION
```

Table 2

CHARACTERISTICS	MIGRAINE	CLUSTER	SMCH†	CONVERSION
MAJOR				
AGE ONSET	EARLY 20's	30	30's	40/s
FREQUENCY	1-3X/MONTH	DAILY	CONSTANT	CONSTANT
DURATION	8-24 HOURS	45 MINUTES	CONSTANT	CONSTANT
INTENSITY	SEVERE	EXCRUCIATING	DULL	SEVERE
LOCATION	UNILAT (80%)	UNILATERAL	BILATERAL	GENERALIZED
ASSOCIATED SYMPTOMS	NAUSEA	LACRIMATION	DEPRESSION	NEUROSIS
	VOMITING	RHINORRHEA		
	PHOTOPHOBIA	HORNER'S		
PRODROMATA	SCOTOMA (10%)			
MINOR				
PAIN CHARACTER	THROBBING	BORING	NON-THROB	NON-THROB
PROVOCATION	ALCOH,STRESS?	ALCOHOL	-	-
MEDICATION USE	PRN	PRN	EXCESSIVE	EXCESSIVE
MEDICAL HISTORY	-	ULCERS(20%)	-	-
FAMILY HISTORY(H.A.)	60%-80%	-	40%-60%	40%-60%

*POST-TRAUMATIC CEPHALGIA IS EXCLUDED FROM THIS TABLE.
†CHRONIC SCALP MUSCLE CONTRACTION HEADACHE

remission period of approximately one year. Each attack lasts between 30-60 minutes and is described as exquisitely severe, always
unilateral, involving the oculo-temporal regions, and associated
with ipsilateral lacrimation, scleral injection, rhinorrhea or nasal
stuffiness, and a partial Horner's syndrome. Attacks may be induced
by alcohol consumption or vasodilators (Ekbom, 1970).

Prodomata, positive family history of cluster headache, or
nausea and vomiting, are not characteristic findings of this
disorder. In chronic cluster headache, remission periods are
lacking.

Chronic paroxysmal hemicrania (CPH) was first described by
Sjaastadt and Dale in 1974. Its major diagnostic features include:
increased headache frequency, eight to fifteen/24 hours; short
lasting attacks, 10-20 minutes; resistance to usual anti-cluster
remedies; and dramatic responsiveness to indomethacin.

Since its existence remains questionable, a discussion of
atypical variants is omitted from this presentation.

Muscle Contraction Headache

Acute Scalp Muscle Headache. Most people will experience
this type of headache under certain conditions. It is likely to
occur during periods of acute emotional, physical, or mental stress.
The headache is described as dull or aching, non-throbbing,
fronto-occipital, occipital, or generalized in location; lasting one
to four hours. Most often, this type of headache is successfully
self-treated with simple analgesics, alcohol, and release from those
stresses initially responsible for the headache.

Not infrequently, an increased pain intensity associated with
the throbbing character may occur, presumably due to a compensating
secondary vasodilatation of cranial arteries. During this phase,
alcohol is contra-indicated while ergotamines are generally
ineffective. Simple analgesics remain the treatment of choice
(Kudrow, 1976).

Chronic Scalp Muscle Contraction Headache. This condition
affects women with a predominance similar to that of migraine. The
mean age of onset, however, occurs a decade later. These non-
throbbing headaches are typically described as constant, always
present, dull in intensity, bilateral in distribution, often fronto-
occipital, in location; and are often associated with neck discomfort, dizziness, and ear fullness.

Moderately severe headaches may occur one to three times a
week, superimposed over the daily, dull headaches. These are often
misdiagnosed as migraine. Such vascular headaches do not respond to
prophylactic anti-migraine medication, but do remit with successful

treatment of the scalp muscle headache component. It probably represents compensatory vascular changes secondary to persistent muscle contraction and increased metabolic requirements.

Many patients claim that chronic scalp muscle contraction headaches are aggravated by tension. A positive family history of migraine in this disorder occurs almost with the same frequency as seen in migraine populations. Chronic scalp muscle contraction headache is most commonly seen in migraineurs, hence the term, combination headache (Kudrow, 1976).

Post-Traumatic Cephalgia

The diagnosis of post-traumatic headache is based on headache onset in relation to a traumatic experience. This may involve accidents in which only minimal or no head injury occurs. Wolff and Simons (1946) had classified post-traumatic cephalgia into three categories. In Type 1, the headache description is indistinguishable from chronic scalp muscle contraction headache. Type 2 is characterized by focal tenderness and pain, superimposed over the Type 1, constant, dull headaches. In our clinic, the criteria for Type 2 has been modified to define Type 1 patients having secondary vascular headache components (Kudrow & Sutkus, 1979).

The Type 4 headache of Vijayan (1977), known as post-traumatic dysautonomic cephalgia, resembles Type 3 post-traumatic headache. Type 4, however, is distinguished by associated features of pupillary dilatation and excessive sweating during the headache attack, and by the presence of an ipsilateral partial Horner's syndrome during headache-free intervals.

Conversion Cephalgia

Severe, constant, non-throbbing or throbbing headaches, causing social and occupational incapacitation for periods of two years or longer, characterize conversion cephalgia. The location of pain is generalized and not associated with nausea or vomiting, unless caused by medication abuse. Aggravation, effort, or responsibilities increase headache intensity.

Typically, the patient appears distant and unaffected as the disabling pain is described. Frequently, a doting spouse accompanies the patient to the doctor's office, eager to interject additional evidence of the patient's sufferings.

Medication abuse is an accompanying feature of the history. A history of migraine precedes the onset of conversion cephalgia in many cases. Traumatic incidents, such as surgery, illness, death in the family, accidents, or injury, may precede the onset of this chronic headache disorder (Kudrow, 1978).

BIOCHEMICAL MECHANISMS IN MIGRAINE

Migraine is considered to be a vasomotor disorder. Even
during inter-headache periods, migraineurs have demonstrated
increased reactivity of blood vessels. Frequently, patients
complain of persistent coldness of hands and feet, especially during
minimally stressful periods. This tendency of peripheral vasoconstriction has been documented (Price & Tursky, 1976). More profound vascular changes have been recorded during the prodromal and
painful stages of classical migraine. O'Brien (1967), and others
(Skinhoj & Paulson, 1969; Norris, Hachinski, & Cooper, 1975; Mathew,
Hrastnik & Meyer, 1976; Sakai & Meyer, 1978), reported that specific
CBF changes occurred during these stages; CBF was found to be
decreased during the prodrome, and increased during pain. Skinhoj
and Paulson (1969) suggested that transient cerebral ischemia was
associated with the prodromal phase of migraine, and approaching
that of carotid occlusive disease. Indeed, Welch et al. (1976) had
demonstrated altered levels of GABA and cyclic AMP in the spinal
fluid of migraineurs, associating these changes to the effects of
ischemia.

Although vascular changes in migraine is of considerable
interest, it is not the primary event in the pathogenesis of
migraine. To this end, one should look at the biochemical events
found to be associated with this disorder.

In recent years, several biochemical pathways of migraine
have been identified. It is not certain whether these biochemical
changes are primary or secondary to this disorder. Nevertheless,
models constructed from these findings help to explain the relationship of environmental influences to the vasomotor changes seen
in migraine.

Serotonin

The importance of biogenic amines in migraine, specifically
serotonin (5-HT), was introduced by Sicuteri et al. in 1961. They
found that during migraine attacks, hydroxyindolacetic acid excretion was increased. This finding stimulated renewed interest in
migraine as a vasomotor disorder, emphasizing biochemical rather
than neurogenic mechanisms.

In 1967, Anthony, Hinterburger and Lance (1967) published a
landmark paper on plasma serotonin changes in classical migraine.
They found that blood platelet serotonin levels significantly
increased during the prodromal stage, and decreased during the
headache phase of migraine. These results confirmed those of
Sicuteri et al. (1967) providing information on the more proximal
serotonin changes associated with migraine attack. Specifically,

Lance, Anthony, and Gorski (1967) showed that serotonin had a strong
constrictive effect on extracranial arteries and, experimentally,
was capable of aborting the migraine attack.

The role of serotonin in migraine was further elucidated by
platelet studies by Kalendovsky and Austin (1975) and confirmed subsequently by Deshmukh and Meyer (1977). The latter authors found
that during the headache-free state, migraineurs showed a significantly lower circulating micro-emboli index and higher aggregability.
Platelet adhesiveness and aggregability increased during the
prodrome, whereas, during the headache phase, adhesiveness increased
significantly, while aggregability decreased. These findings correlated with plasma serotonin changes for both phases of migraine, as
had been demonstrated earlier (Anthony et al., 1967).

Prostaglandins (PGs)

PGs are of considerable interest in migraine, in that they
are vasomotor substances affecting blood vessel changes directly and
indirectly. As has been pointed out by Horrobin (1977), PGE_1, when
injected into non-migraine subjects, caused migraine-like headaches
(Carlsen, Kkelund, & Oro, 1968). As a potent extracranial vasodila-
tor, PGE_1 may cause an internal carotid artery steal, as had been
demonstrated by Welch and his associates (1974) in their innovative
carotid artery blood flow studies on monkeys. Substances known to
influence migraine attacks, such as serotonin, phenylethylamine, and
tyramine, stimulate PG release from the lungs. Further, this
release is inhibited by ergotamines. Sandler (1972) considered this
prostaglandin-release phenomenon an important step in migraine
pathogenesis.

The precursors of PG synthesis are the free-fatty acids.
Prostaglandin endoperoxide is synthesized from arachidonic acid and
in the platelets produce thromboxane A_2 via platelet enzyme
activity. Thromboxane A_2 reduces cyclic AMP levels resulting in a
shape change of the platelets and leads to the release of serotonin,
thromboxane, 5-HT, beta thromboglobulin (BTG), and other substances.
This release reaction is ultimately responsible for platelet
aggregation (Hanberg, Sevensson, & Samuelsson, 1975).

Monoamine Oxidase

Another biochemical marker of migraine is monoamine oxidase,
MAOB, in particular. This is of special interest, since MAOB is a
platelet constituent. In 1970, Sandler and his colleagues (1970)
found an MAOB deficiency in some migraineurs. This study was
prompted by the findings of Hannington (1967), who had documented
tyramine induction in some patients. This suggested enzyme
(monoamine oxidase) deficiency. Subsequently, phenylethylamine oxi-
dizing deficiency was also incriminated in dietary migraine

(Sandler, Youdim, & Hanington, 1974). Sicuteri, Buffoni, Anselmi,
and Del Bianco (1972) reported a platelet MAO deficit in migraine,
confirming the earlier findings of Sandler et al. (1970). Plasma
amine concentrations are increased in the presence of MAOB
deficiency.

Estrogens

Estrogen has clearly a major influence in migraine. Effects
of extrinsic estrogen on migraine frequency have been clinically
observed and documented (Grant, 1968; Whitty, Hockaday, & Whitty,
1966; Kudrow, 1975; Sommerville, 1972).

The mechanisms by which estrogen exerts its influence on
migraine is via its affects on platelet function. Additionally,
estrogens increase plasma anti-plasmin activity, decrease serum
antithrombin activity (Howie, Mallinson, Prentice et al., 1970),
increase platelet aggregability (Mettler & Selchow, 1972), and stimulate prostaglandin secretion directly (Castracane & Jordan, 1976)
and indirectly by stimulating prolactin secretion (Horrobin, 1973).

The Pain Connection

The current concept regarding pain mechanisms of migraine
holds that the site of migraine pain is peripheral. In this scheme,
the initial pathways involve some or all of the biochemical changes
discussed earlier, causing platelet aggregation and serotonin
release, thus inducing cerebral vasoconstriction (the prodromal
phase of migraine). The activation of prostaglandin release from
the lungs by serotonin, and the subsequent depletion of the latter,
causes painful extracranial vasodilatation (the headache phase).
Central serotonin depletion may also lead to a reduced pain
threshold (Figure 1). Fanchamps (1974) includes a second pathway
system that is activated concurrent to platelet release of
serotonin. He suggests that mast cells liberate histamine and proteolytic enzymes. The combined effect of histamine and serotonin
increases capillary permeability. This facilitates transudation of
plasmakinins, formed by the action of proteolytic enzymes on
plasmakininogen, into blood vessel walls and perivascular tissue
(Figure 2). Thus, painful vasodilatation, a lowered pain threshold,
and increased pain sensitivity focally contribute to the migraine
pain.

TREATMENT OF MIGRAINE (TABLE 3)

Treatment consists of three approaches--prophylactic,
symptomatic, and avoidance--and is governed by the frequency,
duration, and severity of attacks. As a rule, patients experiencing
severe headaches more often than twice a month, or having headaches
four days or more per month, are candidates for daily prophylactic

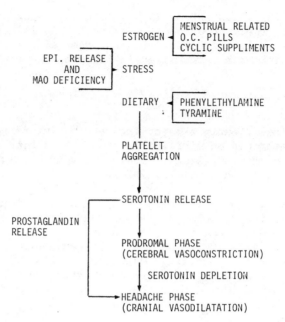

Figure 1.   Platelet aggregation in the pathogenesis of migraine.

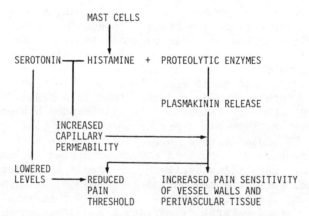

Figure 2.   Mast cell contribution to the pathogenesis of migraine.

measures. At present, the most successful medication available is
propranolol. Initially, the dosage schedule should be 20 mgs.
q.i.d. After one month, or less, it may be increased to 120 mgs. a
day, in divided doses, if significant improvement is not achieved.
Daily doses exceeding 160 mgs. are rarely prescribed at the
California Medical Clinic for Headache.

Table 3

MEDICATIONS	ACTION	CONTRAINDICATION OR CAUTION	MAJOR SIDE EFFECTS
PROPHYLACTIC			
PROPRANOLOL	β-ADRENERGIC BLOCKADE	CONG. HEART FAILURE, BRADYCARDIA,PREGNANCY, PULMONARY DISEASE	OCCASIONAL FATIGUE, RARELY HALLUCINATION
METHYSERGIDE	ANTISEROTONIN	CARDIAC,RENAL,HEPATIC, PERIPHERAL VASCULAR DISEASE, SEPSIS, PREGNANCY, HBP	NAUSEA
CYPROHEPTADINE	ANTIHISTAMINE, ANTISEROTONIN ACTIVITY	ASTHMA,PREGNANCY CARDIAC DISEASE	SEDATION
SYMPTOMATIC			
ERGOTAMINE TART. OR	VASOCONSTRICTOR,CENTRAL	SEE METHYSERGIDE	NAUSEA,VOMITING
DIHYDROERGOTAMINE	α-ADRENERGIC BLOCKER & ANTISEROTONIN ACTIVITY		PARESTHESIAS
ISOMETHEPTENE COMPOUND	VASOCONSTRICTION, SEDATION,ANALGESIA	SEE ERGOTAMINE	LIGHTHEADEDNESS

Propranolol is a beta-blocking agent. Its action on the cardiovascular system results in the lowering of pulse rate, decreasing cardiac output and blood pressure. Because it blocks the action of vascular beta-receptors, the unopposed alpha-adrenergic receptor activity results in an increased vasotonus. This may be beneficial to migraine patients, since extracranial vasodilatation is presumed to be responsible for the pain of vascular headaches. However, it is possible that the major antimigraine action of propranolol is central and not peripheral.

Since bronchospasm is likely to result from beta-blockade, propranolol is contraindicated in patients suffering from intrinsic or extrinsic asthma.

Methysergide, an effective antiserotonin prophylactic agent in migraine, has a rare but unfortunate complication: retroperitoneal and endomyocardial fibrosis (Graham, Suby, Le Compte et al., 1966). This complication may be prevented if, after each three months of daily use, the medication is discontinued for a period of one month. Methysergide is prescribed as a 2 mg. tablet, used 2-4 times per day. Side-effects due to central, gastrointestinal, or peripheral vascular effects may also limit its use.

Symptomatic agents provided to help abort breakthrough attacks are supplemental to prophylactic efforts. Most effective

results are obtained with an intramuscular injection of dihydro-
ergotamine combined with promethazine. The action of the phenothiazine is to prevent nausea and vomiting, while the ergotamine
preparation provides vasoconstriction of extracranial arteries. A
more convenient and only slightly less effective symptomatic treatment consists of the initial use of a promethazine rectal supposi-
tory, followed by oral ergotamine tartrate. Our experience
indicates that the use of ergot in quantities greater than 4 mgs.
per attack does not improve the likelihood of success. Also, the
patient should be cautioned not to use ergotamine more often than
once every ten days, since more frequent use may cause ergotamine-
rebound headaches, greatly increasing headache frequency (Rose &
Wilkinson, 1976). Recent reports also suggest that as little as 7
mgs. of ergot per week is likely to cause asymptomatic, toxic vascular changes (Dige-Peterson, Lassen, Noer et al., 1977).

Recently, biofeedback training has become an accepted modality for treatment of migraine ("Biofeedback," 1978). Indeed, combined EMG and temperature feedback procedures are often used
successfully in this disorder. Children trained in biofeedback
techniques generally show considerably more improvement than do
adults.

PATHOGENESIS OF CLUSTER HEADACHE

Neither etiology nor pathogenesis of this disorder is known.
Numerous investigations have attempted to help clarify these
mechanisms. Horton (1939) concluded, following his initial observation of a number of patients with cluster headache, that external
carotid artery dilatation causes the symptoms of cluster headache
and is mediated by intrinsic blood histamines. He had noted that
during the attack, patients often exhibited enlarged temporal
arteries, relief of pain following compression of the temporal
artery, and ipsilateral flush and skin temperature increase by as
much as $1^{\circ}-2^{\circ}$ c. Contrary to the latter findings, Ekbom and Kudrow
(1979) have not found flushing a characteristic of cluster headache.
In fact, ipsilateral pallor was most frequently observed.

Regarding those changes in the internal carotid artery:
Horven et al. (1972) could find no changes in either the contralateral or ipsilateral internal carotid artery following the placement
of flow meters on these vessels during cluster attacks. Ekbom et
al. (1970) did describe a segmental constriction of the ipsilateral
internal carotid artery in the region of the carotid canal in one
patient having an attack.

An increased intraocular pressure and indentation pulse, as
described by Broch et al. (1970), suggested the possibility of dilatation of the ophthalmic or internal carotid arteries. On Ekbom's
(1970) angiographic study of one patient, dilatation of the

ophthalmic artery was indeed noted.

In a recent study in which we performed Doppler flow and
thermographic examinations, a decreased flow velocity and presumably
decreased flow volume was noted ipsilaterally, suggesting that,
during the attack and interim periods, supraorbital and frontal
arteries were constricted on the side of the headache (Kudrow,
1979).

Anthony (Anthony & Lance, 1971) and Sjaastad (Sjaastad et al.,
1977) independently cited evidence of increased urinary excretion
and blood concentration of histamine in cluster patients when compared with migraine subjects. No changes in serotonin levels among
cluster patients were found in the latter study.

We have shown decreased testosterone and LH levels during the
cluster period and normal values during the remission period among
five cluster patients (Kudrow, 1976). Nelson (1978) confirmed our
results in part, reporting that although mean testosterone levels
were normal in many cluster patients, some had abnormally low values
which could not be explained.

We also found that plasma levels of growth hormone, TSH, FSH,
corticol, T_4, and T_3 were all within normal levels in a small
cluster population (Kudrow, 1980).

Norris et al. (1976) first reported increased cerebral blood
flow values in a patient during a cluster attack. Sakai and Meyer
(1978), in a rather extensive study, presented their CBF findings
from contralateral and ipsilateral hemispheres. During the cluster
attack there was a significant increase in cerebral blood flow in
both hemispheres. However, CBF in the contralateral hemisphere was
even greater than that for the ipsilateral side. CAT-scan examinations and pneumoencephalography in a cluster population revealed no
significant changes, as recently reported by Russell et al. (1978).

TREATMENT OF CLUSTER HEADACHE (TABLE 4)

Prophylactic. The treatment methods for cluster headache
employed at our clinic are based on several considerations,
including age, duration of disease, possibility of medication, and
the presence of other disorders (Kudrow, 1980).

In patients under 30 years of age, prophylactic treatment
with methysergide is recommended. It is less likely to be of benefit at older ages or after having been used for several cluster
series.

Methysergide is prescribed three to four times a day. Most
common side-effects include G.I. symptoms, paresthesias of the

Table 4

CONDITIONS	DRUG OF CHOICE	COMMON CONTRAINDICATIONS AND SIDE EFFECTS
PROPHYLACTIC		
AGE UNDER 30	METHYSERGIDE(2mg,TID-QID)	CARDIAC AND PERIPHERAL VASCULAR DISORDERS,EXTREMITY OR CHEST PAIN,G.I. EFFECTS,PARESTHESIAS
30-45	PREDNISONE(TAPERING OFF FROM 40mg/DAY-3 WEEKS)	ULCERS,DIVERTICULOSIS,HBP, DIABETES,INFECTION
OVER 45	LITHIUM CARBONATE(300mg, BID-QID)	DIURETIC OR LOW SALT THERAPY, TREMOR, G.I. EFFECTS
OTHER ATTACKS IN SLEEP	ERGOTAMINE TARTRATE(2mg,HS)	SEE METHYSERGIDE
SYMPTOMATIC		
	OXYGEN INHALATION, 7L/MIN FOR 15 MIN	NONE
	SUBLINGUAL ERGOTAMINE TARTRATE (1 mg)	SEE METHYSERGIDE

lower extremities, and leg pain. In the presence of such symptoms, discontinuance is recommended. Complications include retroperitoneal, endomyocardial or pulmonary fibrosis, as reported by Graham (1965), Graham and Parnes (1965), and Kunkel (1971). Methysergide is contraindicated in coronary artery or peripheral vascular disease.

Between the ages of 30 to 45 years, it is likely that individuals who had used methysergide for several cluster series have become refractory. Therefore, prednisone prophylaxis is the treatment of choice. Prednisone is prescribed at 40 mg. per day for five days and tapered off over a period of three weeks. It is contraindicated in hypertension, peptic ulcer disease, diabetes, current infection, and in the presence of diverticulosis.

Lithium carbonate, 300 mg., b.i.d. to q.i.d., is our first choice of treatment in patients with chronic cluster (Kudrow, 1977; Mathew, 1978), or in those with episodic cluster (Mathew, 1978), past the age of 45 years. Side-effects are not common after the first day of treatment, before which time G.I. symptoms may occur. In higher doses, tremor is a common side-effect.

Ergotamine is an effective prophylactic medication. In patients who experience one attack daily, 12 mg. of oral ergotamine is provided at least two hours before the expected attack (Kudrow, 1980).

In an earlier study, the effectiveness of prophylactic medication was compared between episodic and chronic cluster groups. In episodic cluster, 77% of patients obtained marked improvement with prednisone. The significant success rate for methysergide was slightly over 50%. In chronic cluster, the most effective results were obtained with lithium carbonate (87%). Prednisone was only 4% effective in this group, and methysergide, 7% (Kudrow, 1978).

Symptomatic Treatment. The most effective symptomatic therapy in either episodic or chronic cluster is sublingual ergotamine or oxygen inhalation. Oxygen at 7 liters per minute for a period of 15 minutes is effective in 70% of patients, 70-80% of the time (Kudrow, in press).

Other modalities of therapy successful in only highly selected cases include indomethacin, cyproheptadine, cryosurgery, nerve or ganglia surgery, and histamine desensitization.

Least efficacious medications or modalities include analgesics, antihistamines, psychotherapy, physical therapy, biofeedback, acupuncture, and manipulation.

DISCUSSION

KUDROW: Yes.

PARTICIPANT: Hi! Dave Gans. I have the same kind of headaches you do. Two questions. One, what's been your experience in the sub-categories of cluster with oxygen for acute attacks? For example, is it as good in secondary chronic as episodic? And the other question is, what's been your experience in the whole family of, a la Raskin, allergic vascular headaches now that people are eating lots of tryptophan?

KUDROW: Well, I don't recognize the category, to answer your last question first, of allergic vascular headaches. I don't know what they are. Then is it still a question? Using tryptophan? Yeah, there were two studies that I remember. In fact, I published one of those studies for someone else when I was editor of the journal and it was an equivocal result and one I did not publish was also an equivocal result. There are no strong studies in migraine with the use of L-tryptophan prophylactically. As far as the oxygen use, your first question, it works just as well in chronic cluster as it does in episodic cluster. And it doesn't matter whether it is primary cluster or secondary cluster. It works well.

PARTICIPANT: Is there any relation between the prevalence of variant angina and the prevalence of cluster headaches?

KUDROW: That's an excellent question. That question has tremendous insight. That's a very good question. Prinzmetal angina is the angina that you're really talking about. There is a relationship. With a person with Prinzmetal, and for that matter, angina secondary to arteriosclerosis decreases, the frequency decreases when they go into their cluster period. John Graham made the association a long time ago and he feels the same pathways that are responsible for Prinzmetal angina are responsible for cluster headaches. Any other questions? Yes.

PARTICIPANT: Regarding the use of either Sansert or corticosteroids in the people with the episodics, how much problem have you had with side effects from the medication?

KUDROW: That's a good question. Methysergide is Sansert and it is a very potent vasoconstrictor. It's contraindicated in people who have cardiovascular, peripheral vascular, or cerebral vascular disease. It cannot be used in people who cannot tolerate the GI effects of that medication also. So you have virtually eliminated about 15% of your potential population, if you wish to use that drug. Now that's the first problem. The second problem is that if they have used Sansert or methysergide for several cluster periods, at some point it will stop working. It's only good for the first few cluster periods. It does not sustain its effect. An intolerance is built up against the Sansert so you are left now with even a smaller population of cluster patients. We usually start methysergide in patients under thirty years of age. Lithium is effective in all patients of all types: episodic and chronic. Cortisone, we do not give to anybody over the age of 45. It has a lot of contraindications too. I don't need to go through all of them for I am sure you know them. But there is one contraindication that a lot of people don't know about and that is diverticulosis. We've testified on two cases now of ruptured diverticular just a few days after starting steroids for cluster headache. And you know the highest incidence of diverticulosis occurs in people over 45 years of age. And since we don't have barium enemas on these people, we routinely do not use steroids in people over 45 years of age. Yes.

PARTICIPANT: I was intrigued in your observation on the data that oxygen would reduce the cluster headache and I just really wondered to what extent, if one did respiratory pattern changes with patients before they have the cluster or during the intercluster episodes, that the headache would disappear. The reason I thought of that, or that I was pleased with your observation, is that the one kind of very chronic cluster patient we worked with who had clusters seemingly two years continuously, if that is at all possi-

ble on a major medication. What we did essentially in a biofeedback
paradigm was shift his breath pattern first and then included also
visualization technique where he would, essentially in his imagina-
tion, blow air right through his eye and in a sense you could say he
is then dilating his internal carotid artery and he became cluster
headache free.

KUDROW: Did you say his headaches were continuous?

PARTICIPANT: They were episodic. He had essentially a chronic
condition of cluster headache and he was out of work for this condition for the two years and then he came to us. Although the
headaches were episodic within that time and he did all the
behaviors. He had the lionized face, excessive smoking, etc.

KUDROW: He was a typical case. When we were halfway through
the study using oxygen in cluster headcache, it was so dramatic that
I immediately got on the phone and I called John Meyer at Baylor and
I told him what our results were and since he has a very good xenon
inhalation blood flow study technique and he also knows something
about headache, I told him very quickly to get the half dozen cluster
patients real quick in the cluster period, give them oxygen and
let's measure their cerebral blood flow. It was an important telephone call because it won him an award for the paper he wrote that
came out of that. In effect, what he showed was that there's a
marked dilation increased, I mean really marked increased cerebral
blood flow in cluster. It is much more than that of migraine. It's
much more than that of anything. Nothing can cause that increased
cerebral blood flow as one sees. However, when oxygen is used,
there's a marked constriction of the vascular bed. There's a massive decrease beyond what one would expect from the effects of oxygen. You know that oxygen is a cerebral vascular constrictor, but
not anywhere to the effect that was observed in cluster headache.
So although studies haven't been done using blood gases, respiratory
changes in terms of oxygen content, and oxygen pressure, we have a
pretty good idea that the relationship has to do with ischemia in
the brain and not a respiratory phenomena.

REFERENCES

Anthony, M., Hinterberger, H., & Lance, J. W. Plasma serotonin
    in migraine and stress. Archives of Neurology, 1967,
    16, 544-552.
Anthony, M., & Lance, J. W. Histamine and serotonin in cluster
    headache. Archives of Neurology, 1971, 25, 225-231.
Biofeedback. Endorsement by the Board of Directors of the
    American Association for the Study of Headache.
    Headache, 1978, 18, 107.
Broch, A., Horven, I., Hornes, H., Sjaastad, O., & Tonsum, A.
    Studies of cerebral and ocular circulation in a patient
    with cluster headache. Headache, 1970, 10, 1-13.

Carlsen, L. A., Kkelund, L. G., & Oro, L.   Chemical and meta-
      bolic effects of prostaglandin E^1 in man.   Acta Medica
      Scandinavica, 1968, 183, 423-430.
Castracane, V. D., & Jordan, V. C.   Considerations into the
      mechanism of estrogen-stimulated prostaglandin
      synthesis.   Prostaglandins, 1976, 12, 243-251.
Dige-Peterson, H., Lassen, N. A., Noer, I. et al.   Subclinical
      ergotism.   Lancet, 1977, 2, 65-66.
Deshmukh, S. V., & Meyer, J. S.   Cyclic changes in platelet
      dynamics and the pathogenesis and prophylaxis of
      migraine.   Headache, 1977, 17, 101-108.
Ekbom, K.   A clinical comparison of cluster headache and
      migraine.   Acta Neurologica Scandinavica (Supl 41),
      1970, 46, 1-44.
Ekbom, K.   Litium vid kroniska symptom av cluster headache.
      Prelininart Meddeland.   Prousc Medica, 1974, 19,
      148-156.
Ekbom, K., & Greitz, T.   Carotid angiography in cluster head-
ache.   Acta Radiologica. Diagnosis, 1970, 10, 177-186.
Ekbom, K. & Kudrow, L.   Facial flush in cluster (Editorial).
      Headache, 1979, 19, 47.
Fanchamps, A.   The role of humoral mediators in migraine
      headache.   Canadian Journal of Neurological Science,
      1974, 1, 189-195.
Goodell, H., Lewontin, R., & Wolf, H. G.   Familial occurrence
      of migraine headache.   Archives of Neurology and
      Psychiatry, 1954, 72, 325-334.
Graham, J. R.   Possible renal complications of Sansert
      (methsergide) therapy for headache.   Headache, 1965, 5,
      12-14.
Graham, J. R., & Parnes, L. R.   Possible cardiac and reno-
      vascular complications of Sansert therapy.   Headache,
      1965, 5, 14-18.
Graham, J. R., Suby, H. I., Le Compte, P. R. et al.   Fibrotic
      disorders associated with methysergide therapy for
      headache.   New England Journal of Medicine, 1966, 274,
      359-368.
Grant, E. C. G.   Relation between headaches from oral contra-
      ceptives and development of endometrial arterioles.
      British Medical Journal, 1968, 3, 402-405.
Hanberg, M., Sevensson, J., & Samuelsson, B.   Thromboxanes, a
      new group of biologically active compounds derived from
      prostaglandin endoperoxides.   Proceedings of the
      National Academy of Sciences of the U.S.A., 1975, 72,
      2994-8.
Hanington, E.   Preliminary report on tyramine headache.
      British Medical Journal, 1967, 2, 550-551.
Horrobin, D. F.   Prolactin: Physiology and chemical
      significance.   Lancaster: Medical and Technical
      Publishing Company, 1973.

Horrobin, D. F. Prostaglandins and migraine. Headache, 1977, 17, 113-117.

Horton, B. T., MacLean, A. R., & Craig, W. M. A new syndrome of vascular headache: Results of treatment with histamine: Preliminary report. Mayo Clinical Proceedings, 1939, 14, 257-260.

Horven, I., Nornes, H., & Sjaastad, O. Different corneal indentation pulse patterns in cluster headache and migraine. Neurology, 1972, 22, 98.

Howie, P. W., Mallinson, A. C., Prentice, C. R. M. et al. Effect of combined oestrogen-progesterone oral contraceptive, oestrogen, and progesterone on antiplasmin and antithrombin activity. Lancet, 1970, 2, 1329-1331.

Kalendovsky, Z., & Austin, J. H. "Complicated migraine," its association with increased platelet aggregability and abnormal plasma coagulation factors. Headache, 1975, 15, 18-35.

Kudrow, L. The relationship of headache frequency to hormone use in migraine. Headache, 1975, 15, 36-40.

Kudrow, L. Plasma testosterone levels in cluster headache: preliminary results. Headache, 1976, 16, 28-31. (a)

Kudrow, L. Tension headache (scalp muscle contraction headache). In Appenzeller (Ed.), Pathogenesis and treatment of headache, New York: Spectrum Publications, Inc., 1976. (b)

Kudrow, L. Lithium prophylaxis for chronic cluster headache. Headache, 1977, 17, 15-18.

Kudrow, L. Comparative results of prednisone, methysergide, and lithium therapy in cluster headache. In R. Greene (Ed.), Current concepts in migraine research, New York: Raven Press, 1978. (a)

Kudrow, L. The enigma of conversion cephalgia. Headache Update, 1978, 2, 7. (b)

Kudrow, L. Thermographic and Doppler flow asymmetry in cluster headache. Headache, 1979, 19, 204-208.

Kudrow, L. Cluster headache. Mechanisms and management. London: Oxford University Press, 1980.

Kudrow, L. Response of cluster headache attacks to oxygen inhalation. Headache, in press.

Kudrow, L., & Sutkus, B. J. Chronic post-traumatic headache: psychophysiolic assessment of minimally-injured patients. Paper presented at the Twenty-first Annual Meeting of the American Association for the Study of Headache, Boston, 1979.

Kunkel, R. S. Fibrotic syndromes with chronic use of methysergide. Headache, 1971, 11, 1-5.

Lance, J. W., Anthony, M., & Gorski, A. Serotonin, the carotid body, and cranial vessels in migraine. Archives of Neurology, 1967, 16, 553.

Mathew, N. T.   Clinical subtypes of cluster headache and
        response to lithium therapy. Headache, 1978, 18, 16-30.
Mathew, N. T., Hrastnik, F., & Meyer, J. S.   Regional cerebral
        blood flow in the diagnosis of vascular headache.
        Headache, 1976, 15, 252-260.
Mettler, L., & Selchow, B. M.   Oral contraceptives and platelet
        function. Thrombosis et Diatheses Haemorrhagica, 1972,
        29, 213-220.
Nelson, R. F.   Testosterone levels in cluster and noncluster
        migrainous headache patients. Headache, 1978, 18,
        265-267.
Norris, J. W., Hachinski, V. C., & Cooper, P. W.   Cerebral
        blood flow changes in cluster headache. Acta
        Neurologica Scandinavica, 1976, 54, 371-374.
Norris, J. W., Hachinski, V. C., & Cooper, P. W.   Changes in
        cerebral blood flow during a migraine attack. British
        Medical Journal, 1975, 3, 676-677.
O'Brian, M. D.   Cerebral cortex perfusion rates in migraine.
        Lancet, 1967, 1, 1036.
Price, K. P., & Tursky, B.   Vascular reactivity of migraineurs
        and non-migraineurs: A comparison of responses to self-
        control procedures. Headache, 1976, 16, 210-217.
Rose, F. C., & Wilkinson, M.   Ergotamine tartrate overdose.
        British Medical Journal, 1976, 1, 525.
Russell, D., Nakstad, P., & Sjaastad, O.   Cluster headache
        pneumoencephalographic and cerebral computerized axial
        tomography findings. Headache, 1978, 18, 272-3.
Sakai, F., & Meyer, J. S.   Regional cerebral hemodynamics during
        migraine and cluster headaches measured by the 133_xe
        inhalation method. Headache, 1978, 18, 122-132.
Sandler, M.   Migraine: A pulmonary disease? Lancet, 1972, 1,
        618-619.
Sandler, M., Youdim, M. B. H., & Hanington, E.   A phenylthy-
        lamine-oxydising defect in migraine. Nature, 1974, 250,
        335-337.
Sandler, M., Youdim, M. B. H., Southgate, J., & Hanington, E.
        The role of tyramine in migraine: some possible bio-
        chemical mechanisms. In A. L. Cochrane (Ed.), Background
        to migraine, Third Migraine Symposium, London:
        Heinemann, 1970.
Sicuteri, F., Buffoni, F., Anselmi, B., & Del Bianco, P. L.   An
        enzyme (MAO) defect on platelets in migraine. Research
        and Clinical Studies in Headache, 1972, 3, 245-251.
Sicuteri, F., Testi, A., & Anselmi, B.   Biochemical investiga-
        tions in headache: Increase in the hydroxyindoleacetic
        acid excretion during migraine attacks. International
        Archives of Allergy, 1961, 19, 55-58.
Simons, D. J., & Wolff, H. G.   Studies on headache: Mechanisms
        of chronic post-traumatic headache. Psychosomatic
        Medicine, 1946, 8, 227.

Sjaastad, O., & Dale, I. Evidence for a new (?) treatable headache entity. Headache, 1974, 14, 105–108.

Sjaastad, O., & Sjaastad, O. V. Histamine metabolism in cluster headache and migraine. Journal of Neurology, 1977, 216, 105–117.

Skinhoj, E., & Paulson, O. B. Regional blood flow in internal carotid distribution during migraine attack. British Medical Journal, 1969, 3, 569–570.

Sommerville, B. W. The role of estradiol withdrawal in the etiology of menstrual migraine. Neurology, 1972, 22, 355–365.

Vijayan, N. A new post-traumatic headache syndrome: Clinical and therapeutic observations. Headache, 1977, 17, 19–22.

Waters, W. E., & O'Connor, P. J. Prevalence of migraine. Journal of Neurology, Neurosurgery, and Psychiatry, 1975, 30, 613–616.

Welch, K. M. A., Chabi, E., Nell, J. H., Bartosh, K., Chee, A. N. C., Mathew, N. T., & Archar, V. S. Biochemical comparison of migraine and stroke. Headache, 1976, 16, 160–167.

Welch, K. M. A., Spira, P. J., Knowles, L., & Lance, J. W. Effects of prostaglandins on the internal and external carotid blood flow in the monkey. Neurology, 1974, 24, 705–710.

Whitty, C. W. M., Hockaday, J. M., & Whitty, M. M. The effect of oral contraceptives on migraine. Lancet, 1966, 1, 856–859.

THE BIOFEEDBACK TREATMENT OF HEADACHES

Jack H. Sandweiss

Director, Sandweiss Biofeedback Institute
Beverly Hills, California

Although clinical biofeedback is currently employed as either a primary or adjunctive therapy in a wide variety of medical problems, it is in the area of functional disorders that the applications and advantages are clear. Since traditional medical approaches to these problems are often temporary and not without side effects, biofeedback offers a viable alternative to the many sufferers of headaches, hypertension, gastrointestinal problems, etc.

Migraine and muscle-contraction headaches represent the largest category of functional disorders seen by most practictioners, yet the development of clinical protocols for these problems is still in its infancy. Furthermore, the study of biofeedback approaches to headache, given their diverse patterns and combinations, provides heuristic value by serving as a model by which to view the biofeedback treatment of functional disorders in general. Therefore, although this chapter will focus upon biofeedback and headaches, the basic philosophy of the treatment plan is applicable to many other problems of somatic dysfunction and is best understood in terms of the conceptual model put forth by Gary Schwartz (1977). That is, biofeedback intervention ultimately involves the alteration of patterns of central neurogenic processes through the use of instruments which monitor relevant parameters of organ behavior. Although the exact mechanisms by which these alterations come about are yet to be understood, the expansion of clinical biofeedback into other functional areas is currently limited by the state of the art of non-invasive, continuous recording technique. However, the current availability of both sensitive feedback thermometers and EMGs provide a means for altering physiologic behavior which is relevant to migraine and tension headaches in large numbers of patients.

The employment of biofeedback techniques in the management of

both migraine and tension headaches is best viewed in the context of
biofeedback approaches to pain problems in general. Although much
has been said about biofeedback and the relief of pain, its relevance is clear only under the following two circumstances: when the
pain is due to a physiologic dysfunction which can be altered by an
appropriate biofeedback modality, such as pain associated with acute
muscle spasm or claudication pain; or, when the pain, or its underlying cause, is either triggered by or exacerbated by stress, which
is often the case with back pains, arthritic pains, irritable bowel
syndromes, etc.

One of the fascinating aspects about studying biofeedback and
headaches is that these pains often demand a dual approach. That
is, a few migraines and many tension headaches appear to be due to
an underlying physiological propensity to respond inappropriately to
stressful events or situations. Furthermore, it is important to
remember that with regard to measurable correlates of subjective
pain, normative data does not exist and would only have clinical
relevance if transformed into a score that took into account the
apparent wide differences in pain thresholds. Thus, absolute EMG
levels and peripheral temperatures often fail to correlate with subjective pain experiences across patients. On the other hand, small
relative changes in these parameters often produce dramatic clinical
results.

Before discussing protocols, I would like to point out that the
practice of clinical biofeedback is currently governed by no legal
authority, and there are no enforceable clinical standards. The
varieties of experiences that patients encounter in biofeedback
clinics borders on the ludicrous. Some "biofeedbackers" leave their
patients alone for an hour attached to instruments and listening to
a tape recorder. The therapist returns after sixty minutes to
collect the fee. Others, would you believe, don't bother with the
instruments, but they call it biofeedback anyhow. Therefore, please
accept the following remarks as only regarding one way of doing biofeedback which has evolved over the last several years as a result
of my working with patient populations in hospitals, universities,
and the private clinic which I direct.

First of all, out-patients who are treated for somatic complaints such as headaches are accepted only upon diagnosis and
referral from physicians who are following the patient for the disorder. Furthermore, all treatment plans are individualized with
respect to modalities employed, homework assigned, and number of
treatment sessions. Our patients are not run through a standardized
stress reduction program. Although session length is usually one
hour and frequency is typically once per week (that's the way the
world works), our patients are now receiving longer and more frequent initial sessions which taper off as progress is made. These

kinds of decisions, however, are always arrived at by mutual agreement between the therapist and the patient.

INTAKE

Sometimes the entire first session is devoted to intake, and the necessity of an intake process that is oriented toward the development of an appropriate biofeedback treatment plan is a point that I would like to underscore. At our clinic, the biofeedback therapist always contacts the patient by telephone in order to arrange the first appointment, and the therapeutic value of this initial interaction is realized. First impressions are important, and the respect shown by the therapist for the patient's problem, which is usually briefly discussed at this time, can often bias the sessions to follow in either a positive or negative direction.

Upon arrival at the initial session, patients are asked to provide demographics and complete a simple stress questionnaire. Psychological tests and inventories such as the MMPI and MCMI are not routinely administered to nonpsychiatric patients, for it is our experience that such instruments provide little, if any, information of value in designing an appropriate biofeedback treatment plan. Furthermore, insistence upon such testing as part of a standardized intake process often alienates the patient, because the patient senses no face validity to what he is being asked to do. Thus, obligatory psychological testing for patients who perceive only somatic complaints runs the risk of damaging the therapeutic relationship from the beginning, and offers little if anything to gain. The remainder of the first session consists of a personal interview by the therapist followed by an explanation of our methods to the patient. Physiological feedback is usually initiated before the end of the first hour.

The therapist has more than one task to accomplish during the initial session with an overall goal of getting to know the patient. How does the patient spend her day? Is she the kind of person who would practice breathing exercises at work? What would be the best terminology to use in explaining biofeedback to this patient? Answers to these kinds of questions are imperative if one is to design a realistic treatment plan, that is, one based upon a rationale appropriate to the disorder, and one that the patient will follow. Lack of motivation on the part of patients is often traceable to a lack of creativity on the part of the therapist, and this becomes an even more challenging problem in asymptomatic disorders, such as most cases of hypertension.

The second intake task which we find necessary is that of validating the diagnosis. Particularly in the area of differential headache diagnosis, there exists widespread confusion and a lack of definition. Migraines can be mild or severe, unilateral or bilat-

eral, accompanied by nausea or not. Over the years they have been
called by a number of contradictory descriptors such as summer headache and winter headache, vacation headache and washday headache
(Dalessio, 1972). Furthermore, many migraine headaches have tension
headache components and some patients experience alternation between the two types with an occasional sinus headache from time to
time, which can make diagnosis very confusing. Therefore, we retake
the medical history from the beginning, and, if there is any question of agreement with the diagnosis, our medical director reviews
the case. If necessary, the matter is resolved with a telephone
call to the referring physician.

DIFFERENTIAL DIAGNOSIS

     Regarding the differentiation between migraine and tension
headaches, the key discriminators from a clinical standpoint appear
to be the presence or absence of prodromal signs and the patient's
response to medication, ergot derivatives in particular. So-called
classic migraines are relatively easy to define by the presence of
preheadache phenomena. The difficulty comes in distinguishing common migraine from tension headache. And, since many of these
patients have combined headaches with both vascular and muscle contraction components, sorting out the etiologies of the various head
pains is not easy. However, a distinction between common migraine
and tension headache can often be made from an examination of the
medical history of the patient. The response of the headache to
vasoconstrictive agents as compared to the response of the headache
to non-narcotic analgesics and muscle relaxants often sheds much
light on the nature of the underlying dysfunction. In other words,
if a headache can be aborted by sublingual ergot taken at onset, or
relieved by ergot IV after becoming well-developed, then it is most
probably of vascular origin. On the other hand, if the pain can be
eliminated with aspirin, Fiorinal, or Valium, and is not helped by
vasoconstrictors, then a tension headache diagnosis is more likely.
Also, tension headache patients typically exhibit elevated EMG
levels in the posterior neck and shoulder regions and often complain
of recurrent neck pain and stiffness. Although tension headache
pain patterns tend to be both frontal and suboccipital while
migraines tend to be more temporal and parietal, location of pain is
not a significant discriminator in our experience.

TREATMENT

     Once the interview portion has been completed, the process of
biofeedback as well as the rationale underlying the treatment to
follow is carefully explained to each patient in a manner to which
he or she can relate. Our experience overwhelmingly supports the
notion that virtually all patients, regardless of their backgrounds,
can understand the physiological natures of their problem, and the
reason for biofeedback, if both are properly explained. This kind

of patient education clearly enhances treatment outcome, because now
the sessions have meaning to the patient, and that in turn increases
patient motivation. Fahrion, in his work with hypertensives, also
finds patient education to be a relevant clinical factor (personal
communication). Motivational issues are even more difficult in
asymptomatic disorders, but these problems should not be looked upon
as deficiencies in the patient. Instead, they should be accepted as
challenges to those practicing biofeedback to develop creative
solutions. Following the intake process, physiological feedback is
begun and the first modality employed is based upon diagnosis. A
clinical hypothesis of migraine almost invariably leads me to begin
with peripheral temperature training, but before examining the
protocol, I would like to present the rationale for this approach
which is based upon the following model.

As illustrated in Figure 1, the gradual buildup of vasoconstrictive activity brings about the perception of an "aura" when
ischemic conditions along branches of the internal carotid arteries
reach a hypothetical threshold. In the absence of any intervention,
these vascular changes rebound into a vasodilatory "head pain" phase
which primarily involves branches of the external carotid. If vasoconstrictive agents, such as derivatives of ergotamine tartrate,
are taken at the onset of the aura stage, the normalization of the
relevant cerebral vessels takes place as the result of the combined
action of vasoconstriction (due to the ergot) acting upon a homeostatic rebound mechanism.

On the other hand, vasodilatation through learned sympathetic
reduction at the onset of the aura also normalizes the relevant
vessels by aborting the vasoconstrictive buildup prior to the rebound stage. Thus, the irony of both a chemical vasoconstrictor and
a behavioral vasodilatation technique producing the same result is
explained by the model. It is important to remember that the aura
can take many forms; it is sometimes simply a feeling of impending
headache.

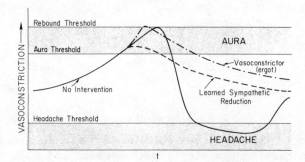

Figure 1. Functional Model of Classic Migraine.

    When the patient learns voluntary reduction of sympathetic
activity and brings it about prior to the rebound, the aura disappears and no headache follows in 70 to 80% of patients in clinics
around the country, using various kinds of instrumentation and
different definitions of migraine. The most common way of accomplishing this is through teaching handwarming, but handwarming
should not be confused with learned sympathetic reduction. If the
hands warm up and the feet cool off, has sympathetic activity been
reduced? Those who routinely observe foot temperatures note absence
of correlation between hand and foot temperatures while handwarming.
And, what about heart rate? The point that I am trying to make is
that generalizations about sympathetic activity in general cannot
be made from changes in a single gross record of vascular behavior.
In some individuals, EMG-assisted relaxation is necessary in addition to peripheral temperature training in order to bring about
changes necessary to avoid migraines. The coupling that must exist
between these and other peripheral measures with the central mechanisms responsible for migraine has yet to be discerned, because
there is still no easy way to monitor cerebral vascular changes non-
invasively. Those who suffer from common migraine achieve similar
results by practicing learned sympathetic reduction periodically,
thus preventing the vasoconstrictive buildup in the first place.
This might parallel the use of Propranolol, a beta-blocker, as maintenance therapy for common migraines. Again, the model would pre-
dict that any method of preventing vasoconstrictive activity from

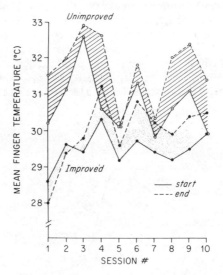

Figure 2. Note. From "Peripheral temperatures in migrainers
undergoing relaxation training" by M. Werbach and J. H. Sandweiss,
Headache, 1978, 18(4), 212. Copyright 1978 by Headache. Reprinted
by permission.

building up could be useful in aborting migraines, and this is
illustrated in Figure 2. In this study, 45 migraine patients
entered a program of biofeedback-assisted relaxation training.
Relaxation methods employed included hypnosis, meditation, autogenic
training, etc. Peripheral temperature training was specifically not
taught, although peripheral temperatures were monitored throughout.
Of the 37 patients who completed ten training sessions, 27 (74%)
were rated as improved. A significant inverse correlation was found
between the ability to warm hands during the first session and
treatment success. Although patients who improved showed increased
hand temperatures across training sessions, the gain scores were not
significant. In other words, the migraine relief appeared to be due
to general relaxation training, as opposed to the specific ability
to warm hands (Werbach & Sandweiss, 1978).

However, learned sympathetic reduction, when effective, has a
number of advantages over other migraine therapies, in that it is a
brief, low cost therapy, with side effects that are almost always
beneficial. It is also interesting to note that many classic
migraine patients notice a reduction of preheadache signs and subsequent headaches after they have aborted a few migraines. In other
words, they no longer practice learned sympathetic reduction and
they remain asymptomatic. It appears that their bodies have learned
something. I would now like to move to a discussion of muscle contraction or tension headache.

These are best described as the result of elevated skeletal
muscle activity in the muscles of the neck, shoulder, jaw, forehead
or scalp, and the pain is often referred as well as local. For the
purpose of appropriate protocol selection, these individuals can be
classified into several groups. The largest category includes those
who respond to routine stresses in their lives with inappropriate
tightening of the relevant musculature. Therapy is directed toward
identifying the relevant stresses and areas of tension by extensive
interviewing and multi-site EMG monitoring. The success of this
approach depends upon how well the therapist can help the patient
transfer either specific or general EMG relaxation to his or her
daily life. It is explained to these patients from the beginning
that coming to the clinic once a week and relaxing in our recliner
for an hour is not going to accomplish anything and that our homework instructions must be followed or treatment will be discontinued. Our experience also indicates that tension headaches, in
particular, tend to involve patterns of responding that are inextri-
cably linked to one's lifestyle, and, therefore, cannot be modified
without parallel lifestyle alterations. Once again, patient resistance to such changes is greatly lessened by therapists who take
whatever time is necessary to explain carefully the interaction between lifestyles, stresses, and headaches to the patient. Once the
patient has an understanding of the possible etiology of the problem
and the rationale for biofeedback, then compliance with homework

becomes less of an issue.

Homework for these patients consists of both periodic and random muscular relaxation excercises. Random exercises are those
triggered by unpredictable daily events, such as a ringing telephone. They must occur at a moderate frequency, five to ten per day
in order to retain their effectiveness. They must be individualized
to a patient's lifestyle and daily routine. But, they serve the
dual function of both interweaving appropriate responses into the
patient's daily life, and offering a barometer by which patients can
observe their own progress. After a while, if things are working
properly, the appropriate muscles are already relaxed when the random cue occurs. The reinforcing aspects of this last point should
not be overlooked. With regard to homework, the therapist explains
to each patient at intake that successful integration of learned
physiological control depends upon practicing specific exercises
without instruments. These assignments can vary tremendously
because they have got to be matched to the patient's lifestyle and
personality. Unrealistic demands that are not met are counter-
therapeutic, so all decisions regarding homework should be arrived
at and agreed upon mutually. Some of our patients do exercises that
last thirty minutes, and others practice thirty seconds at a time
when that is felt to be appropriate.

Sometimes, elevated EMG levels in patients are not caused by
phasic responses to stressors, but are brought about and chronically
maintained by improper breathing, that is, the utilization of
accessory breathing muscles, in particular the upper trapezius and
sterno-mastoid, while inhaling at rest. This inappropriate habit,
instilled in Western men and women for cosmetic reasons, has been
responsible for large numbers of tension headaches in our patient
population. Biofeedback provides a simple method for correcting
this habit and teaching diaphragmatic breathing. First, it is
determined whether the patient suffers from chronic pulmonary problems, because their presence adds doubt to the wisdom of this procedure. Those patients with reduced lung efficiency may simply need
the assistance of upper chest and neck muscles in order to achieve
sufficient lung volume, and, in these individuals, insistence upon
diaphragmatic breathing can quickly lead to a futile situation which
does the patient no good. In appropriate patients, however, the
correction of improper breathing can dramatically eliminate headaches due to this habit within three to four weeks. This procedure
involves having the patient practice EMG-monitored diaphragmatic
breathing while sitting in a straight-backed chair and utilizing
home exercises designed to generalize this practice into the daily
routine. EMG monitoring of accessory breathing muscles with the
patient in different postures offers an objective index of the
degree of recruitment of the inappropriate musculature. Keep in
mind that when first learning to breathe in this manner, it is
usually much easier in a supine position and considerably more dif-

ficult while standing. Therefore, we initially use multi-site EMG monitoring with the patient in different positions, in order to determine the optimal initial posture. This should be a posture that offers a moderate challenge, and as progress is made, the position is changed with the goal of teaching the patient proper breathing in a standing position. It is very important to remember that visual observation of neck and shoulder movements while practicing breathing is no substitute for multi-site EMG recording, since some individuals isometrically tighten these muscles while inhaling and there is no visible indication that they are breathing improperly. Homework for these patients consists of three exercises which I have found to be extremely effective at turning around breathing patterns in a short period of time. The first one consists of repeating at home the practice that is learned in the office, i.e., practicing deep diaphragmatic breathing while sitting in a straight-backed chair. The second exercise consists of lying on a hard surface (like the floor) and practicing pushing up a ten-pound weight which is placed on the abdomen. This exercise has the effect of strengthening the abdominal muscles and teaching the patient the proper rhythm of breathing. The third exercise consists of a random event, like a ringing telephone, triggering a body inventory of how one is breathing at the moment. This latter exercise is designed both to weave correct breathing into a patient's daily routine, and to serve as a barometer of improvement. It is explained to all patients that they might feel some transient muscle soreness as abdominal muscles are stretched for the first time in many years.

In those situations where the headaches are solely due to improper breathing, they stop occurring as soon as the patterns are corrected. Sometimes, only partial symptom reduction is noticed and additional work is needed. When that happens, the residual headaches are dealt with anew as a remaining component of a combined headache. Although the term "combined headache" normally refers to headaches with both muscle contraction and vascular components, some muscle contraction headaches can have parallel causes, as in the case of headaches aggravated both by chronically elevated upper trapezius tension and nocturnal teeth-grinding in the same patient.

Finally, a small minority of tension headache patients has chronically elevated upper chest, shoulder, and neck tension because they are psychologically defending themselves against the world with their bodies. Many of these people report that they find themselves holding their breath throughout the day. It is not always easy to identify these individuals at intake. Usually, they exhibit a variety of negative feelings and emotions when almost any kind of relaxation technique is employed, and, when such characteristics are observed, biofeedback is stopped and the patient is reevaluated from a psychological perspective. Even if one is a skilled therapist, the rapidity with which biofeedback has been known to strip away

somatic defenses must be respected. In these patients, biofeedback
is clearly not recommended as a primary treatment modality, but can
have value as an adjunct to an ongoing psychotherapeutic relationship.

INSTRUMENTATION

It is amazing that even though instrumentation is the singular
distinguishing feature between biofeedback and all of the other
self-control techniques, there are still debates over its necessity.
I also find it interesting that those who minimize their importance
often refer to them as "machines," which they certainly are not, and
which is a misnomer that carries the connotation of an active
process, unlike most of today's biofeedback. So, for the record,
machines perform work and instruments record. I believe that the
words are important because when a patient hears that he is going to
be attached to a machine, he rightly assumes that something is going
to be done to him and may be subsequently disappointed. This can
obviously interfere with his assumptions and expectations about the
first session, and need not happen in the first place. Furthermore,
it is the instrumentation that allows us to operationalize dependent
variables. This is necessary in order to build the kind of data
base that biofeedback is building, totally unlike the other self-
control techniques. This means that biofeedback protocols are amenable to statistical determinations of efficacy, again unlike the
other self-control techniques. Clearly, the use of instrumentation
must be a part of any definition of biofeedback, and the utilization
of instrumentation accounts for many differences between biofeedback
and the other methods.

Now, during the period when physiological feedback is being
given, the advantages of instruments which combine sensitivity and
accuracy with interesting and creative feedback displays cannot be
overstated because they help the therapist make the sessions more
meaningful and enjoyable. Patients who stop showing up for biofeedback sessions when they know that they will be listening to the same
tone going slowly up and down for another hour are not lacking in
motivation. The treatment protocol has simply extinguished any that
they might originally have had. It is also important to remember
that the goal is self-regulation, and once a patient has acquired
the skill necessary to bring about the desired physiological change,
external feedback is rapidly diminished, but physiological monitoring continues for a while just to make sure.

REINFORCEMENT

When instruments are used optimally, their value as reinforcers
is maximized. Since the role of reinforcement in clinical situations is seldom discussed, a brief review is appropriate. Remember,
all reinforcements are rewards, and they can be positive when some-

thing, like money, is added to someone's environment, or negative when something undesirable, like a splinter, is removed from someone's environment. Both positive and negative reinforcements are rewards. In the operant conditioning work out of which biofeedback grew, the reinforcement was imposed on the animal with electrical stimulation to the medial forebrain bundle and other pleasure centers. With people, that cannot be done and the situation is far more difficult and complicated. However, as Finley's work with cerebral palsy children indicates, appropriate positive reinforcement leads to lower dual site EMG recordings than standard lights and sounds (Sandweiss, 1978). The children were rewarded with pre-selected toys from a vending machine triggered by low and constant EMG levels according to a pre-set criteria, and they achieved far lower EMG levels than with standard types of audio and visual feedback.

Reinforcement with adult patients presents a far more difficult problem, and their toys are a lot more expensive. It is the task of the therapist to understand and utilize the patient's value system, not the therapist's, in arranging the reinforcement contingencies. The therapist must realize that the personal interaction between him or her and the patient is extremely relevant from an operant point of view. Of course, acquiring the skill and symptom relief have obvious reinforcement value, but it is the therapist who shapes and mediates the process. Direct verbal reinforcement by the therapist based upon physiological information known to both is far more motivating to most people than moving a needle or lowering a tone. And, as in all medical therapies, a receptive and confident practitioner adds to the overall atmosphere of the treatment and enhances compliance with homework, thereby increasing the probability of a successful outcome.

REFERENCES

Dalessio, D. J. Wolf's headache and other head pain. New York: Oxford University Press, 1972.

Sandweiss, J. H. (Ed.) Handbook of physiologic feedback (Vol. 4). Berkeley: Pacific Institute, 1979.

Sandweiss, J. H. Vascular disorders in biofeedback. In UCLA Fundamentals of biofeedback, Los Angeles: Center for Integral Medicine, 1978.

Werbach, M., & Sandweiss, J. H. Peripheral temperatures in migrainers undergoing relaxation training. Headache, 1978, 18(4), 211-214.

THE MULTIMODALITY MANAGEMENT OF HEADACHES

Lee Kudrow, William H. Rickles, and Jack H. Sandweiss*

RICKLES: I would like to approach the topic of multimodality
management of headaches in terms of control because that is the term
today. We could have said therapy and so forth, but control is the
common word now. Control or treatment. One can think of approaches
through environmental control, psychosocial stress control, ANS
(autonomic nervous system), stress response control or specific
pathophysiological control. These are the three areas. Now briefly
to go through these. For example, under environmental control:
one, there may be factors having to do with the weather, physical
trauma, foods, allergens, or society in general. Obviously, a
therapeutic approach to these would be education and perhaps avoid-
ance. You might want to leave this society and go to another one or
leave where these particular antigens originate and go to another
area or whatever. Under psychosocial stress control there's the
possibility of teaching interpersonal coping, assertion training,
stressor identification, psychotherapy, behavior therapy. A wide
variety of methods can be used to approach the interpersonal coping
to control stress at the psychosocial level. Or one might approach
this from an intrapsychic rather than sociological or interpersonal
way. There's the intrapsychic coping capacity, such as cognitive
restructuring methods or psychodynamic psychotherapy or psychoanalysis, for example. ANS stress response control, systematic
desensitization, or relaxation therapy, general biofeedback therapy,
some of the body therapies, physiotherapy, or some of the more
unconventional alternative body therapies or drugs. A variety of
ways to approach this level of control of the psyche soma disorder.
And finally, specific pathophysiological control, there are the biobehavioral therapies: that is biofeedback, specific biofeedback

*See List of Contributors for addresses.

aimed at a specific pathologically reacting system such as hypertension or physiotherapy. And then of course drugs. Drugs that act specifically on acute symptomatic therapy, such as the ergotamines in migraine headache, or prophylactic therapy, such as Inderal, propranolol. I think now we would call this a systems approach. Various systems can be approached. Perhaps some day it would be possible to make an evaluation, a total person or holistic evaluation of a patient at each of these levels. One may conceive of other levels also. And what contribution difficulty or dysfunction at each level may make to the final common pathway of the symptom of the disordered soma and then structure the intervention according to that assessment. So I think I just wanted to present these slides to start off the concept of the multimodality approach to a psychosomatic disorder and in this case to headache. And see what my other fellow panel members, Dr. Kudrow and Mr. Sandweiss, may have to say about multimodality approaches and any questions that you may want to put to any of the three of us.

PARTICIPANT: Rick, I'd like to ask you, since you began with this notion of multimodality therapy. I think you have to take it one step further. Give me some rules for deciding which one to begin with, how to know to stop one, and start another, how to deal with the interactions among them. It's nice to say these and it's like God, country, and motherhood. One couldn't argue with it. But one needs to take it a little further than that.

RICKLES: We published a paper a few years ago about the biofeedback treatment of a woodwind musician who had tics and various problems. We treated him with EMG feedback and negative and positive practice and so forth and it was a very successful case. A point that we made in the discussion of this patient was that if you just look at him as a person who has tics and can't ply his trade as a woodwind musician, you would miss the point and you would also probably not be successful because before we ever got to the point of giving him biofeedback training, his utterly chaotic family life, his problem with alcohol and so forth, had to be dealt with first. I think that at the present time that comes under the heading of clinical judgment and assessment of a more complete situation. Yes, of course, it is God, motherhood and the flag and apple pie and, uh, Inderal for the headache's effect, that would be in there too, but sometimes we need to say it again and, in the direction of getting the quantitative evaluation, begin to set it down in a specific way. That's what I was attempting to do, of course, but I don't think I can go into how to assess each of one of those individually. That's part of our work for the next fifty years.

PARTICIPANT: I don't want to anticipate paragraph 12 of my talk tomorrow. (laughter) What's a psychosomatic disease?

RICKLES: I'm going to tell you about that Sunday. (general

laughter)   I have a whole hour to tell you about what a psychosomatic disease is this Sunday.

PARTICIPANT: I would like to hear from Dr. Kudrow on multimodalities.

KUDROW: I hope you don't want to hear about psychosomatic
disease from me; I haven't used that term in about 15 years.   I'm
not sure about this multimodality form of therapy.   Headache is a
very narrow field, a very narrow speciality, and I've had the good
fortune of being very interested in a very narrow field.   I've con-
centrated all my efforts on just a small discipline without having
to worry about what else was going on around the world of medicine.
And because of this, you know, intense concentration in this limited
area, we have evolved, in our clinic, certain notions, certain
ideas, that I would like to pass on to you.   Where one would consider multimodalities would be in certain headache disorders and
certainly not in other headache disorders.   Disorders that may indicate the need for multimodality therapy would include chronic scalp
muscle contraction headaches, I'll define that for you, post-
traumatic headaches, and there are four types of those, and conversion cephalgia.   Now clinically, chronic scalp muscle contraction
headache is very easy to diagnose.   Now I hope that doesn't contra-
dict Jack Sandweiss' earlier statement where he felt that there was
some difficulty in diagnosing between chronic scalp muscle contraction and migraine.   We don't seem to have that difficulty.   Chronic
scalp muscle contraction headache simply is headaches that occur
daily.   It's constant: you wake up with it; you go to bed with it;
and it's dull in intensity, fluctuating, day in and day out, every
day, all day, all the time for many years.   We use a minimum criteria of two years.   If they have it for longer than that, they fit
in the criteria.   One doesn't need more than that because there virtually are no other types of headache conditions that imitate that.
If you see someone who has these constant dull headaches for a
period of longer than two years, it's chronic scalp muscle contraction headache.   Now, how do these people score on psychometric
texts?   Uh, poorly, not terribly, but poorly.   Some of them have
conversion Vs.   What they have on scales one and three are significantly elevated, with a dip in scale two.   They seem to have a
suppressed depression, you might say.   They are hysterical, and
they're somewhat hypochondriacal.   Going on to the next worst type
of headache would be the post-traumatic cephalgia, and I'm specifically talking about post-traumatic type one.   These are people who
present virtually the same as chronic scalp muscle contraction headache people.   The only difference is they had an accident that preceded their headache onset.   They score grossly abnormal on MMPIs.
Very specific.   We did the study two years ago.   It's been cross-
validated by two other studies since.   The last one is yet to be
published in Headache.   These people have these constant dull headaches.   They're somewhat incapacitated in terms of their depression.

They are poorly responsive to medication. They're difficult to evaluate because of the litigation status that occurs in many of these people, and they score a little worse on their MMPIs than do the chronic scalp muscle contraction headache people. They have elevations in scales 7 and 8; there seems to be a rise in the schizophrenic scale. The worst of all the headache disorders are the conversion cephalgia headaches. Constant, day in day out for many years. These people are socially and occupationally incapacitated. They usually come into an office with a doting spouse who very often hands out the pills to them, describes to you their pains if the patient has missed anything. It's a syndrome. They have all of these characteristics in common and one of the most important characteristics of the conversion cephalgia is the apathetic faces, the belle indifference. The patient will be describing this excruciating, constant pain the way I'm talking to you now. They score grossly abnormal on the MMPIs. Very high schizophrenic scale, high on 7, very low on introversion scale, and of course, elevation in scales 1, 2, and 3. Virtually 6 or 7 out of the ten scales are abnormally high. These people are very easy to distinguish from . . . in fact, each headache disorder is, in fact, not hard to distinguish. Now, how are these people treated by us? Chronic scalp muscle contraction headache people . . . about 70% respond dramatically, and I mean dramatically, to amitriptyline. Not so much imipramine, but amitriptyline. It appears one needs a serotonergic effect that amitriptyline has. They are both norepinephrine sparing, but also amitriptyline has a serotinergic effect which appears to be the source of the success. Two and one half, three weeks after they start the medication, just as with depressive patients, the headaches start to go away. One does not need to get into the massive doses of amitriptyline that one does when they're treating depression. Twenty-five mg., 35 mg., 50 mg. can be sufficient. Quite a bit different from depression patients. Posttraumatic patients only do half as well as chronic scalp muscle contraction patients with amitriptyline and there's a question of whether there's litigation neuroses interfering with their success. Conversion cephalgia patients do not do well. Conversion cephalgia people are untreatable. We've had success in something like five out of 200 patients. And one of the major problems is they're medication abusers. It's not unusual for someone to be taking 30 aspirin a day or 30 fiorinal a day or a combination of 30 aspirin and 30 fiorinal a day. We saw one patient who took 100 aspirin a day and that's not to mention the barbiturates that they use or the narcotics that they use and it's impossible to wash them out. They won't go into the hospital; they won't participate in the multimodality thing by seeing a psychiatrist or a psychologist; they simply won't participate. They'll get bored with biofeedback and leave after the third session. They're unhelpable. But a multimodality approach would be wonderful, if they would cooperate. But when you talk about chronic scalp muscle and post-traumatic, it's unnecessary to have multimodality approach. One can simply use the medication, amitriptyline, that works best. And in combination with biofeedback, the success rate is even higher. Nina Matthew just published on that.

SANDWEISS: Sometimes we've noticed that . . . of course psychological changes will come along, or one level of change, will come along when another level is worked on. A couple of years ago, I treated a physician who had terrible migraine headaches that were sensitive to ergot, but it was very difficult for him to take ergot preparations. It was a very complicated situation. As a matter of fact, diuretics were sufficient for him to abort the migraines, but we didn't have any success at all in biofeedback, and then about six months later, he phoned me and he said, "You know, we have a slight history of epilepsy in our family so, just for the hell of it, I started taking phenobarb," and what happened was that the headaches stopped and, more importantly, his whole personality changed. He was far less obsessive/compulsive, which one might expect, if you're on a slow, long-acting barbiturate. But I think a lot of times you can effect change in one level by working on the other, at least from my point of view, because my assumption is that they're all really looking at the same thing. That it's all essentially chemical and that even the psychotherapeutic relation or psychotherapeutic treatment, when it is successful, would have to have correlative chemical changes.

PARTICIPANT: I have two questions. One, for Dr. Kudrow. If you have success using Inderal as a prophylactic against migraine headaches, do you still go on to pursue something like biofeedback to avoid any possible . . . or not?

KUDROW: That's a very good question. We have found, as others have, that a combination of biofeedback and medication works better than either alone.

PARTICIPANT: But, do you try to get rid of the Inderal altogether, or would you still stay with some level of Inderal?

KUDROW: It's very hard to get rid of medication. See, migraines spontaneously disappear providing there's no iatrogenic interference. As an example, giving patients estrogen after they reach menopause . . . they usually disappear post-menopausally and it's unnecessary at that point to maintain them on medication. But if patients are having frequent migraines for a number of years, they'll require prophylactic medication for a number of years.

PARTICIPANT: The other question I have was for Mr. Sandweiss. You mentioned the lack of efficacy to a certain extent when you only monitor one item in terms of monitoring central nervous system sympathetic discharge, for example, temperature in the finger. Is there experimental work now that uses multi . . . or at least is attempting to get multi-dimensional monitoring and further, is there any clinical work being done with that kind of approach?

SANDWEISS: I believe I was referring to the fact that biofeed-back, because of the instrumentation, allows us to operationalize variables and that's what allows for statistical determinations of efficacy. With regard to the second question, I think it should be done. The only one I'm really aware of doing it in a systematic way with hypertensives is Steve Fahrion, where he's combining hand and foot warming together, but I think that the possibility of doing the two with say throwing in heart rate or something like that would give a lot clearer indication that overall sympathetic activity was reduced. The study that was mentioned this morning, by the way, that appeared in Biofeedback and Self-Regulation, again, utilized a single, sympathetic measure and the authors concluded, in my opinion fallaciously, about things going on in the sympathetic system as a whole.

PARTICIPANT: What study was this?

SANDWEISS: There was a question this morning . . . there was an article in Biofeedback and Self-Regulation, a "careful double blind study." In the last paragraph of that article, the authors admit that there are a number of methodological problems with their study, and there have been problems with others. I think one of the things that happens a lot is that many studies have a control and experimental group, and the control groups sit quietly as if that's no treatment, and yet if one interprets "sitting quietly" as any kind of relaxation, then once again, there's a clear reason for what's going on, they're reducing sympathetic activity. And if you want to call that a placebo, fine, but I think that that hides what might really be happening in those cases.

PARTICIPANT: I'm trying to understand the connection between sympathetic activity and migraine headache. What has sympathetic activity got to do with a migraine? What is the postulated mech-anism, in other words, if you warm a hand, what are you doing to the migraine? And why is that some people under stress conditions do not get migraine whereas when they are "relieved," where one might assume there is less sympathetic activity, the migraine breaks through? I just don't understand the whole thing.

SANDWEISS: Well, the connection, I think, is just simply that migraines are vascular and sympathetic branch of the ANS controls vascular flow.

KUDROW: Migraine is considered to be a vasomotor disorder. The vasomotor system is under the control of the autonomic nervous system. The sympathetic nervous system is one part of the autonomic nervous system, in part, regulated by the hypothalamus. So,

migraine is, you might say, a sympathetic nervous system disorder.
Now, Matthew (not Nina, but Roy Matthew), from Texas, did a very
interesting study recently and I don't think it's published yet, but
it will be shortly. They drew catecholamine levels and they did a
number of things. In fact they did EMG measurements as well as
drawing catecholamines on patients before biofeedback and after biofeedback. And they did several other things that I don't remember.
There was a marked drop in catecholamine responses. They also
measured, if I'm not mistaken, the monoamine oxidase, and there was
a marked increase in monoamine oxidase after biofeedback. You know,
nobody really knows. I don't think anyone here could answer, "What
does biofeedback do?" It's obviously doing something more than we
can explain. But that is true for all of medicine. You know, nobody can explain anything. We just have to work at it bit by bit
until it comes together.

PARTICIPANT: Well, gentlemen, what do you do with a classic
hypochondriac? I had a lady, 48, who has had chronic TMJ pain.
She's had three surgeries, been in and out of the hospital, I think
six times, for a variety of complaints, most of which they can find
no organic etiology for. She has made 12 appointments in my office
for biofeedback, you know the TMJ relaxation thing, just to see what
would happen. She has broken six of ten appointments because she
hurts so badly she can't come in from twenty miles away. Her husband says her mother and sister and her sister-in-law all have
psychosomatic complaints of one kind or another and have had all
their lives. Yet her mother is 88 years old and still feeling
miserable. Do you have any comments on the TMJ thing?

KUDROW: I think this is the type of patient that I mentioned
earlier. These are the patients with the doting husbands, etc. We
cannot help them. Quite simply, we've tried everything. We have to
wait for medical science to progress, and new things to be found
out, before we could approach them successfully. If anyone else has
any idea, I'd like to hear . . . something from the floor? God
knows, that's not why I'm up here.

JACOBS: I think this afternoon for the first time it hits me
how vague is this notion of control of sympathetic outflow. And I
really am not so much asking a question as making an observation
that may form a good basis for discussion. One of the things that
seems to me to be fairly clear is that there are real idiosyncratic
but specific ways that people respond to stress which would imply
that it's not a generalized sympathetic outflow even within the
visceral system, let alone whatever connections you have to CNS
mechanisms, and that there are very specific kinds of trained mechanisms at work here producing the disorder. And the notion that what
we are doing is reducing the generalized tone of sympathetic outflow
and thereby producing an effect, seems to me to be a little bizarre
unless the intention of that notion is that we're doing something

about making a generalized biochemical change, for example, in MAO
levels, etc., which then would have some further effect. But to
argue that a specific physiological effect is being produced by
something called a change in generalized sympathetic outflow,
strikes me as just too vague and probably incorrect. I mean out
flat incorrect, empirically. So there. (laughter)

SANDWEISS: I totally agree, Dave.

PARTICIPANT: I wanted to respond to Dr. Kudrow's question
about the lady that was just mentioned with TMJ syndrome and suggest
that as a clinical lifesaver in cases like this and my reasoning
goes as follows: first, what I would do with that lady, I'd put her
on amitriptyline and don't ask me why, but I would in a minute.
About 150 mgs. a day, and she'll probably never wake up from it,
will be the response. Secondly, what I would do is I would look to
myself, 'cause I do it all the time and we all do it as physicians
and the dynamic comes like this: somebody walks into the office and
says, "Finally, after all these years, I've found you, and you're
gonna fix me, aren't you?" You say, "I'm pretty groovy. I'm gonna
fix you." And then you're doomed, O.K.? You're not gonna fix her.
And she doesn't want to be fixed and so the response to that is,
"No, you have a syndrome the best I can figure out has 75% response
rate if you come in and do the biofeedback this many sessions for
this much time and if you do the exercises at home." And when she
says, "But I hurt too much or I can't come in or that's not enough
magic," then what you have to say is "Tough, isn't it?" And that's
all you can say, but you are not responsible for fixing her. She is
responsible for fixing her with biofeedback, which is a different
dynamic than if I give you a pill and say "I will fix you." Then I
have taken on the responsibility for fixing you in a slightly different way. Haven't I? And then I am liable to that response,
that's O.K., it's good for my ego, but I would like to sidestep it
with patients like this 'cause it's not gonna work.

ENGELS: I don't want to respond specifically to your question
because I haven't had that kind of clinical experience. I just
haven't. But I do know that there is a moderate literature on this
that is worth exploring. I mean it's not just a case of faith
healing and testimonials. There is work, and the person I think
who's most, who has done the most work in this area is a man named
Barry Blackwell, who developed a psychosomatic service when he was
at Cincinnati and carried it to Dayton and is now at Mt. Sinai in
Milwaukee where he developed, I think, reasonably effective programs
for dealing with patients whom he called patients with multiple
somatic complaints. I know that one aspect of his argument is that
you must redefine the concept of treatment and not treatment. If
you expect cure in the usual medical sense, then that's not going to
work. These are patients, who have had a long history of using
these multiple somatic complaints reasonably effectively and the

reason they're so effective is because if you manage one, then
they'll just develop another. And these are the people that end up
in surgeon's hands very often because they keep looking until
finally they find someone who will cut them. And if you don't make
the referral, then they'll just move on to another doctor who even-
tually will. But I would urge those of you who are interested in
the problem to look at Blackwell's writings.

BIOFEEDBACK IN PHYSICAL MEDICINE AND REHABILITATION

Steven L. Wolf

Associate Professor, Department of
Rehabilitation Medicine
Assistant Professor, Departments of
Anatomy, Surgery and Community Health Sciences
Coordinator, Biofeedback Research Programs
Emory University School of Medicine
Atlanta, Georgia

INTRODUCTION

Muscle, or electromyographic (EMG), biofeedback refers to the use of electronic instrumentation to make covert muscle activity obvious to the patient through the display of visual and auditory representations of muscle contractility from within the pick-up radius of surface or indwelling electrodes (Wolf, 1978). This form of feedback is used by many practitioners engaged in relaxation training to reduce hyperarousal behavior. Under most circumstances in which general relaxation is sought through application of EMG biofeedback, the magnitude of change in measurable integrated muscle activity is comparatively small, often under 20 uV (microvolts). On the other hand, when muscle biofeedback is applied to patients with specific musculoskeletal or neuromuscular pathologies, appropriate sensory-motor functions and hence, coordinated and meaningful movement patterns, require electromyographic changes often exceeding hundreds of microvolts. In addition, unlike the results from feedback applications designed to re-establish homeostatic mechanisms within other physiological systems (for example, improve peripheral blood flow or systolic-diastolic differentials or alter heart rate), muscle biofeedback produces outcomes that are obvious even to the casual observer. Thus, while feedback of a cardiovascular activity might improve psychophysiological measures related to hypertension, often the attainment of self-regulatory control is unappreciated by clinician or patient. Feedback to re-educate abnormal movement behavior, however, will always result in a functional behavior that

83

is visible and easily quantified. Invariably, these elements contributed to the prediction by Fernando and Basmajian (1978) that, with respect to physical rehabilitation, "EMG feedback techniques will become routinely used" and ". . . EMG biofeedback has provided a major impetus for the advance of our body of knowledge for treating neurological dysfunctions."

Why should EMG biofeedback permit substantial functional improvement to occur among chronic neurological patients whose conditions have stabilized or remained unresponsive to conventional rehabilitation procedures (Brudny et al., 1979; Wolf, Baker, & Kelly, 1979)? The application of any neuromuscular facilitatory technique designed to re-educate weakened or paralytic muscles usually necessitates interfacing the clinician between stimulus and response. Following a command or instruction, the clinician observes the patient or palpates an appropriate body segment. Immediately following the patient's response, the practitioner assesses performance and "feeds back" a verbal instruction to the client. At best, this sequence takes a few seconds and, even when a premiere clinician evaluates a patient's movement activity, her subsequent command is comparatively non-specific.

On the other hand, muscle biofeedback provides continuous, uninterrupted and precise information about muscle activity delineated by the pick-up area of recording electrodes and by the properties of the feedback equipment (that is, signal-to-noise ratio, amplification, etc.). Therefore, specificity of the content and immediacy of the feedback distinguish machine from clinician, and for learning (or relearning) of any motor skill ongoing cerebral processing of activity, also called knowledge of results is essential (Howson, 1976). The central nervous system's remarkable capacity for processing audio and visual representations of muscle activity in a meaningful temporal and spatial manner to ultimately improve sensory-motor integration probably accounts for the success of this modality among many rehabilitation patients.

The primary purpose of this presentation is to review the development of EMG biofeedback in rehabilitation from both historical and clinical perspectives so that the practitioner can better appreciate the observations just noted. Secondary purposes underlying the relevance of this article are to describe other forms of feedback (force and positional) presently employed in the rehabilitative process and to address future needs and directions to more appropriately comprehend the importance of these electronic devices.

HISTORICAL PERSPECTIVE

The predecessor of what is today known as muscle biofeedback was first described by Marinacci and Horande (1960). These clinicians used an electomyogram to provide "feedback" of raw muscle

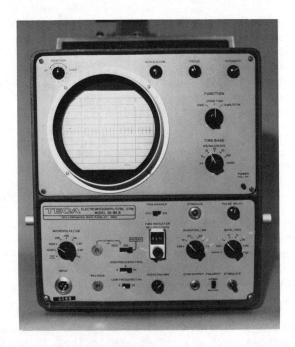

Figure 1. Clinical electromyograph used to perform EMG biofeedback.
Raw EMG signals appear on oscilloscope screen. Knobs on front panel
control sweep speed of trace across the screen and gain or magnifi-
cation of muscle potentials. Muscle responses are shaped by changing
the gain.

potentials from an oscilloscope screen (Figure 1). Audio feedback
was conveyed by use of an audio amplifier. The task for each
patient was simply to retain the peak-to-peak amplitude of raw EMG
signals between two consecutive horizontal divisions on the electromyograph screen. By adjusting the "gain" or amplification of the
voltage signal from muscle potentials, the clinician could make the
task easier or more difficult. For example, to strengthen a
weakened muscle, the gain (sometimes called "sensitivity") would be
continually lowered so that more effort would be necessary to produce muscle potentials whose peak-to-peak amplitude would span one
horizontal division. This technique is analogous to what is today
known as "shaping" responses. The electromyograph is still used by
many clinicians as a feedback device as well as an instrument from
which one can evaluate muscle potentials for possible pathology.

At the same time, researchers (Harrison & Mortensen, 1962;
Basmajian, 1963) were learning that, given appropriate visual and
auditory cues, man, could learn to isolate and control single motor
units in most voluntary skeletal muscles. In fact, the ability to

perform this unique motor skill was in no way related to specific
psychosocial attributes (Basmajian, 1974). It must be remembered
that a motor unit consists of a single motor axon, its terminal
branches and all the muscle fibers supplied by those terminals.
Indeed, the demonstration that man could control these discrete
neurophysiological entities in the absence of activity from the
remainder of a muscle was definitive proof of our remarkable capacity for finite movement.

    The information in Figure 2 demonstrates that a single motor
unit isolated from the medial gastrocnemius muscle can be significantly influenced by subtle changes in vertical posture. Note that
every time the patient is slightly tilted toward 90 degrees (full
upright position) at about a 70 degree angle from the horizontal
position, motor unit activity increases. While these motor units
are easily controlled in normal individuals, their occurrences in
spastic muscle are more frequent than previously thought (Regenos &
Wolf, 1979) and actually may impede efforts toward relaxation in the
presence of EMG feedback.

    The numerous demonstrations of single motor unit control sum-
marized by Basmajian (1974) actually preceded the advent of contem-
porary EMG feedback; yet served as the logical transitional phase
between kinesiological electromyographic analyses and muscle

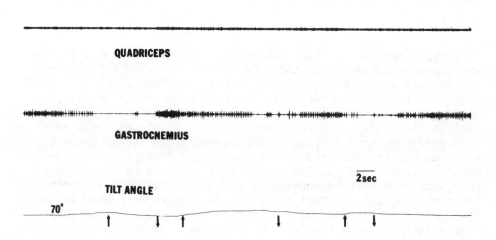

Figure 2. Single motor unit isolated from medial gastrocnemius
muscle. This unit increases frequency with subtle adjustments in
angle of tilt table about 70 degrees from horizontal (downward
arrows, trace 3). Trace 1, EMG from quadriceps; trace 2, EMG from
medial gastrocnemius; trace 3, angle of tilt table.

biofeedback clinical techniques. If man, in other words, could isolate and control motor units in the presence of visual and auditory
representations of that activity, then certainly patients demonstrating neuromuscular dysfunction could use similar "feedback" from
entire muscles or muscle groups to alter abnormal or weak movement
patterns. It was within this context that the first EMG biofeedback
clinical reports emerged (Booker, Rubow, & Coleman, 1969; Jacobs &
Felton, 1969; Amato, Hermsmayer, & Kleinman, 1973; Johnson & Garton,
1973; Brudny et al., 1974).

MUSCULOSKELETAL APPLICATIONS

When the central nervous system is intact, patients will have
very little difficulty using feedback signals to effect changes in
muscle strength or force. In most cases, the situation is one in
which muscle output must be increased because of weakness following
limb immobilization or orthopaedic surgery. Perhaps the relative
simplicity of interfacing patient to machine accounts for the few
published reports (Napliotis, 1976; Sprenger, Carlson, & Wessman,
1979; Wolf, 1980) demonstrating facilitation of improvement and
reduction in rehabilitation time when muscle biofeedback is integrated within an exercise or electrical stimulation treatment program for muscle weakness or joint instability.

Figure 3 shows the basic operating principles to strengthen the
quadriceps femoris muscle following knee surgery. Recording electrodes are first placed very closely together over the rectus
femoris muscle of the quadriceps group (Figure 3A). The sensitivity of the feedback device is set quite high so that even the
slightest contraction localized in the proximal portion of the
muscle will be detected and fed back to the patient. With
increasing volitional effort, the patient attempts to increase the
tone from the audio amplifier or the dial deflection of the feedback
device (Figure 3, background). Once accomplished, the sensitivity
of the machine is reduced so that the patient must contract the
muscle even further to receive feedback of similar magnitude to that
provided at a lower sensitivity setting. In the process, the
patient invariably recruits more motor units from the quadriceps
mass. The entire procedure is repeated several times, but with
progressively wider reference electrode placements (Figure 3B-D).
Using this protocol, patients are often capable of developing full
isometric contractile force within two treatment sessions.

A similar strategy is employed in treating patients with peripheral nerve injuries, provided that electromyographic evidence of
reinnervation is present. We have had extensive experience treating
patients with Bell's palsy (Brown et al., 1978) using EMG biofeedback to weak facial muscles. The primary strategy centers about
increasing EMG activity from a weak muscle without overexaggerating
activity from the unaffected side. Invariably, two threshold feed-

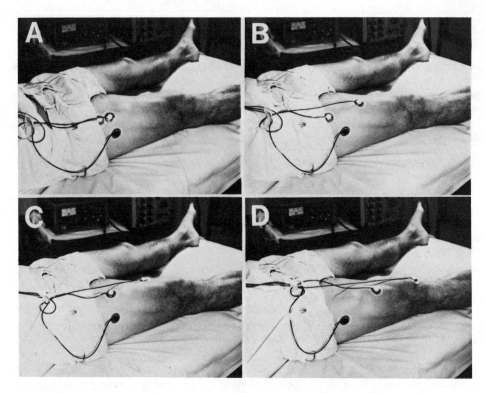

Figure 3. Reference electrode placements used to recruit more
activity from quadriceps muscle following knee surgery. Reference
electrodes are white snaps and ground is black snap. Note progressive separation of reference electrodes in A-D as more muscle activity is sampled. Feedback unit in background (Reproduced with
permission from Wolf, S.L. Electromyographic biofeedback in exercise programs. The Physician and Sports Medicine, 1980, 8, 61-68.)

back units are used; one is set to provide audio feedback to weak
muscles when the integrated EMG activity exceeds a pre-set level,
while the other audio tone is given when integrated EMG levels from
the "strong" side also exceed a threshold level which is set comparatively low. The patient strives to activate the former but not
the latter tone. Visual feedback is provided from a mirror. An
additional constructive task requires the patient to activate only
the threshold feedback from the weakened muscle or muscle group as
he attempts to read aloud with exaggerated lip and facial musculature movements.

EMG biofeedback applications are also amenable to a host of

tendon or muscle transfer techniques to facilitate learning use of
the transposed muscle. A bizarre example of this application
involves specific training of the gracilis muscle (adductor muscle
of the thigh) using closely spaced electrodes. The patient learns
to increase EMG output from this muscle, which is subsequently
stripped in longitudinal fashion. Half the muscle remains in place
while the other half is detached from its insertion at the medial
aspect of the knee and threaded into a circular configuration within
the pelvis as a new external anal sphincter. This bisection can be
accomplished because of the multiple endplate arrangement of the
gracilis (Coers & Woolf, 1959). Following surgery, the patient
learns to contract the reconstructed anal sphincter through additional feedback given to the remaining half of the gracilis within
the thigh. Our success in implementing this feedback procedure has
been recently confirmed by other investigators (Berrol et al.,
1980).

Additional applications of EMG biofeedback for musculoskeletal
retraining await on the horizon (Wolf, 1980). For years the
Japanese and East European countries have assessed electromyographic
activity patterns from elite athletes as a basis for training young,
aspiring competitors. These novices are trained to stimulate the
temporal and spatial muscle activation patterns recorded from
acknowledged "superstars." It would appear reasonable to speculate
that telemetered EMG could be interfaced with a feedback mode to
inform the athlete when his movement or muscle pattern is optimal;
that is, provide feedback, based upon previous analyses, as the athlete actually performs. The immediacy of this feedback has obvious
benefits over post-hoc assessments of performance from videotaped
replays.

NEUROMUSCULAR APPLICATIONS

Applications of EMG biofeedback to patients with cerebrovascu-
lar accidents (stroke) have received more attention than applications to other disorders affecting the central nervous system.
Numerous controlled clinical studies (Basmajian et al., 1975; Lee
et al., 1976; Middaugh & Miller, 1980; Hurd, Pegram, & Nepomuceno,
1980; Binder, Moll, & Wolf, 1981) attest to the viable potential for
EMG biofeedback to help restore neuromuscular function, either as a
separate treatment entity or as an element within a comprehensive
exercise program. In total, however, data from these investigators
have been contaminated by our continuous efforts to group stroke
patients together without considering the specific central locus of
pathology and consequent clinical problems, such as receptive or
expressive aphasia or dyskinesia. As a result, specification
regarding the types of stroke patients most amenable to treatment
with EMG biofeedback is lacking. Development of single case study
designs (Gianutsos et al., 1979) will invariably contribute to
clarification of the most important training components for

successful muscle re-education among stroke patients using this
modality.

Despite these limitations, outcome studies among chronic stroke
patients have been encouraging. Published data clearly indicate
that improved function following feedback training can be attained
(Brudny et al., 1976; Basmajian, Regenos, & Baker, 1977). In our
own work (Wolf, Baker, & Kelly, 1979) we have demonstrated that,
with stringent criteria, patients are able to make remarkable gains
in function, with approximately 60% learning to ambulate independently and 30% gaining full use of the upper extremity. These
patients were considered complete successes (Table 1). One year
comprehensive follow-up data obtained through detailed neurophysiological measurements indicated that none of the patients with success or moderate grades (Table 1) had regressed (Wolf, Baker, &
Kelly, 1980). Therefore, sensory-motor integrative skills resulting
from feedback training appear to have been learned.

Primary deterrents to improvement appear to be related to the
severity of proprioceptive loss. The age or sex of patients, duration of stroke or previous rehabilitation and side of the cerebral
lesion are not correlated with outcome. Data relating duration of
stroke to number of biofeedback treatments or duration of previous
rehabilitation for all outcome grades are depicted in Figures 4 and
5, respectively. As can be seen in these figures, successful treatment of the lower extremity of hemiplegic patients could be achieved
at any time following stroke, while success in treating involved
upper extremities tended to occur among stroke patients within 50
biofeedback sessions (Figure 4), and primarily when these patients
had received less than one year of previous rehabilitation (Figure
5).

Table 1

Outcome Grades and Criteria Following EMG Biofeedback

Training Among A Chronic Stroke Population

Grade	Criterion
Success	Complete functional use of limb for activities of daily living.
Moderate	Change in neuromuscular status associated with functional gains.
Failure	No change or some change unassociated with functional gains in neuromuscular status.

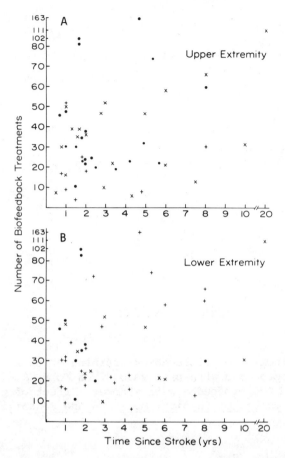

Figure 4. Outcomes for biofeedback training of upper (A) and lower (B) extremities of chronic stroke patients. Abbreviations: +, success; ., moderate; x, failure (as defined in Table 1). Abscissa is in time since stroke for A and B. (Reproduced with permission from Wolf, S.L., Baker, M.P. and Kelly, J. L. EMG biofeedback in stroke: Effect of patient characteristics. Archives of Physical Medicine and Rehabilitation, 1979, 60, 95-102.)

Training stroke patients to improve in neuromuscular abilities involves adhering to specific treatment strategies that we have developed for the upper (Kelly, Baker, & Wolf, 1979) and lower (Baker et al., 1977) extremities. Essentially, these strategies center about reduction of activity in spastic muscles followed by recruitment of muscle responses in weak, antagonist muscles. This training proceeds in a proximal to distal direction. For upper extremity training, the patient begins in a supine position and sub-

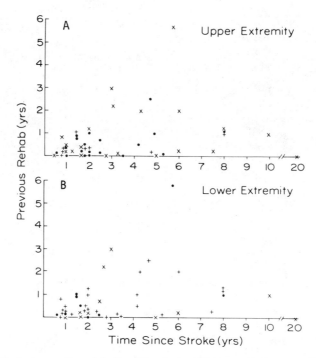

Figure 5. Outcomes for biofeedback training of upper (A) as in
Figure 4. (Reproduced with permission from Wolf, S.L., Baker, M.P.,
& Kelly, J.L. EMG biofeedback in stroke: Effect of patient charac-
teristics. <u>Archives of Physical Medicine and Rehabilitation</u>, 1979,
<u>60</u>, 95-102.)

sequently repeats the training sequence in sitting and standing
postures. During lower extremity biofeedback applications, the
patient position progresses from sitting to partial weight-bearing
to full weight-bearing. Ultimately, improvement is assessed through
quantified neuromuscular and functional measures. Although much of
our recent data collection is still in the analytic phase, it would
appear that the single most important factor in predicting improvement with this modality is not the amount of muscle activity the
patient learns to generate, but rather his ability to inhibit
hyperactivity from spastic musculature during induced stretch or
lengthening contractions of these muscles.

     Considerable interest has been expressed in the use of EMG bio-
feedback for the treatment of patients with incomplete spinal cord
injury (SCI) and some preliminary data appear encouraging (Owen,
1974; Schneider et al., 1975; Seymour & Bassler, 1977). In our
own experience using EMG biofeedback to treat paraplegic patients

with incomplete spinal cord injuries, we have found that this modality is effective in training patients to reduce the occurrence and intensity of lower extremity muscle spasms. This goal is achieved by training patients to relax specific muscle groups both at rest and during passive stretch of muscles from which spasms emanate. Only after patients are able to achieve this end do we initiate feedback training to increase muscle activity voluntarily. Many of our patients claim that their ability to control muscle spasms while simultaneously reducing or eliminating drug therapy promotes increased function by allowing them to attend to specific activities without interruption. Whether patients will progress with EMG biofeedback to ambulate either independently or with assistive devices for longer distances and periods of time remains to be seen.

In training cerebral palsy patients with EMG biofeedback, questions have arisen concerning long-term maintenance of measured short-term improvement (Skrotzky, Gallenstein, & Ostering, 1978) or carry-over to untreated limb segments (Spearing & Poppen, 1974). Reduction in EMG activity recorded from facial muscles appears to parallel improvements in speech and motor function (Finley et al., 1976). Positional feedback has also been effective in helping these patients to gain control of head-to-body orientation (Wooldridge & Russell, 1976). Yet, specific clinical training strategies have not been resolved for interfacing cerebral palsy patients with EMG biofeedback. Much of these patients' abilities to improve motor function depend upon their intellectual levels and carry-over capacities. In our own experience we have found that young cerebral patients are capable of reducing activity in hypertonic leg muscles when a variety of feedback alternatives is provided to them. These youngsters invariably become bored with the novelty of feedback and new methods must be developed to maintain their concentration and interest. One device that has proven effective in our hands has been the bioconverter (Brown & Basmajian, 1978). This device provides feedback when the integrated EMG recorded from a specific muscle moves beyond a pre-set threshold level. Any alternating current device plugged into a power source will be activated when muscle activity exceeds a threshold level. By plugging a radio, television, or carousel with consecutive slides into the power supply, the young patients will work to maintain input from any one of these appliances. This procedure allows us to maintain interest among our cerebral palsied clients.

Within the past several years, EMG biofeedback techniques have been employed in the treatment of patients with chronic low back pain. The general premise underlying the use of biofeedback has been the reduction of excessive activity from paraspinal muscles by combining the feedback with relaxation training techniques. The presumption has been that muscles of the low back are excessively active. This notion has met with some resistance. Indeed, not all patients with chronic low back pain have exaggerated muscle activity

(Wolf et al., 1979). Two patients with similar diagnoses may show completely opposite electromyographic activity levels from spinal musculature at rest. What has become apparent to us, however, (Jones & Wolf, 1980) is that invariably chronic back pain patients show asymmetrical patterns of muscle activity from each side of the back during simple movements such as forward bending and lateral rotation with the pelvis stabilized. Our training strategies, therefore, have been developed to assist patients in producing equilibrated muscle activity from both sides of the vertebral column. This procedure involves the simulation of movements which exacerbate pain on the part of the patient while paraspinal muscles are analyzed from biomechanical perspectives for their appropriate responses. Patients are then trained to change responses that approach what would be expected as normal. In essence, these patients are undergoing a procedure designed to teach them to inter-nalize their conceptualization of postural readjustments. To date, our initial results with this training procedure appear encouraging. Apparently, in our experience, there is no one single procedure that can be used universally for all chronic low back pain patients when EMG biofeedback is the primary treatment choice.

Several years ago my colleagues at Emory University recognized that patients receiving EMG biofeedback for increased finger joint mobility following repair of lacerated finger flexor tendons were capable of generating vast amounts of muscle activity without improving mobility of the affected joint (Kukulka, Brown, & Basmajian, 1975). As a result, finger electrogoniometers were con-structed as feedback devices. Initially, these goniometers resembled those developed by Long and Brown (1964) for kinesio-logical investigations. Our electrogoniometers were modified so that a potentiometer placed at the base of the goniometer could pro-duce a voltage change proportional to the change in a variable resistor as the potentiometer was moved. This movement, in turn, when exceeding a specific voltage change, could activate an audio amplifier, thus providing feedback to the patient. By further incorporating a threshold within the feedback device, activation of a tone would become contingent upon exceeding a certain degree of joint mobility.

Since that time, our joint positional feedback goniometers have undergone considerable revision. Our group has constructed numerous goniometers for wrist and hand joints (Brown, DeBacher, & Basmajian, 1979). One such example is depicted in Figure 6. This particular electrogoniometer is designed to provide feedback as the patient moves the wrist into further extension. The potentiometer is located at the proximal base of the electrogoniometer. Input from the potentiometer is led to an audio amplifier (Figure 6, Metal Box), where a tone is emitted when the patient exceeds a predeter-mined increase in wrist extension. The electrogoniometers are made of lightweight plastic and are extremely durable. These goniometers

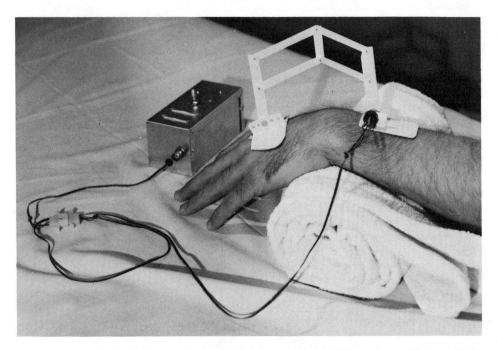

Figure 6. Wrist electrogoniometer interfaced with audio amplifier
(left). Potentiometer with lead wire is placed proximally. (Reproduced with permission from Wolf, S.L. Electromyographic biofeedback
in exercise programs. The Physician and Sports Medicine, 1980, 8,
61-68.)

can be constructed cheaply and weigh less than 10 grams.

Electrogoniometers are extremely beneficial to signal increased
joint mobility in combination with functional electrical stimulation, to improve joint movement following contractures, and to
facilitate coordinated movements of patients suffering from central
nervous system deficits. For example, we frequently combine electromyographic and joint positional feedback to improve wrist and finger
function. This procedure involves providing a patient with two
feedback tones. On the one hand the patient must maintain activity
in the spastic wrist and finger flexor muscles below the specified
level while simultaneously working toward increased wrist and finger
extension through goniometric feedback. The goal in this situation
is to maintain silence from feedback monitoring the wrist and finger
flexors and induce feedback from the joint goniometer as wrist or
finger extension is achieved.

Recently we have developed a pronation-supination feedback

device. Since the muscles which supinate (palm up) the wrist are
located deep within the arm, surface electromyographic biofeedback
is not practical. Similarly, the muscles which pronate (palm down)
the wrist, while superficially located in the forearm, are very
close to the muscles which flex the wrist. As a result, despite
placing electrodes close to one another on the skin surface, flexor
activity may be recorded. The device shown in Figure 7 is designed
to substitute positional feedback for electromyographic feedback.
The rod placed along the dorsal aspect of the forearm simulates the
course of the radius bone. A potentiometer is anchored with straps
over the approximate location of the head of the radius. The distal
end of the rod is curved and placed over the styloid process of the
radius. As the forearm is pronated and supinated the rod turns
within the potentiometer and produces a voltage change proportionate
to a change in a variable resistor housed within the potentiometer.
When movement exceeds a predescribed number of degrees, an audio
tone from the device shown to the left in Figure 7 is activated.

FORCE FEEDBACK APPLICATIONS

     The device depicted in Figure 8 is a feedback cane (Baker,
Hudson, & Wolf, 1979). A series of strain gauges placed along the

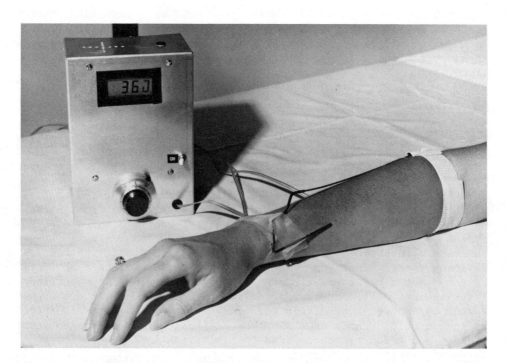

Figure 7.   Pronation-supination positional feedback device placed on
dorsal forearm. See text for details.

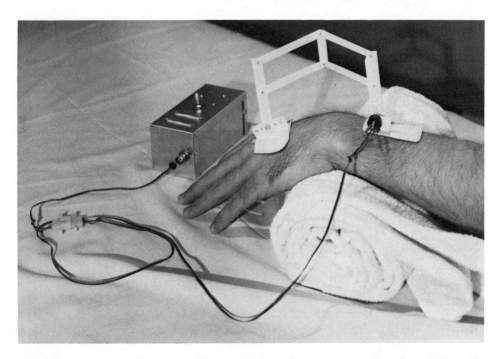

Figure 8.   Feedback cane connected to audio amplifier.   See text for details.

shaft of the cane signal forces applied through the handle.   When these forces exceed a predetermined level set by the hand-held device, an audio tone is emitted.   This particular feedback cane was devised for patients with receptive and expressive aphasia for whom verbal instructions provided little benefit during the rehabilitation process.   By simply attending to the presentation of a tone, these patients quickly learn to shift weight from the cane to the opposite lower extremity.   As this process progresses, the threshold is set lower so that a tone will be emitted with less force through the shaft of the cane.   This shaping procedure helps to train patients to shift weight onto an affected lower extremity, thus becoming less dependent upon the use of an assistive device for ambulation.

Wolf and Hudson (1980) have modified the Krusen Limb Load Monitor to help patients improve gait.   The original limb load monitor is represented by the force plate (foreground, Figure 9) and the audio amplifier (left rear, Figure 9).   The force plate is placed within a shoe.   When the force through the insert exceeds a predetermined level, an audio tone is emitted.   Our modification can be seen in the upper right of Figure 9.   Since patients bear weight

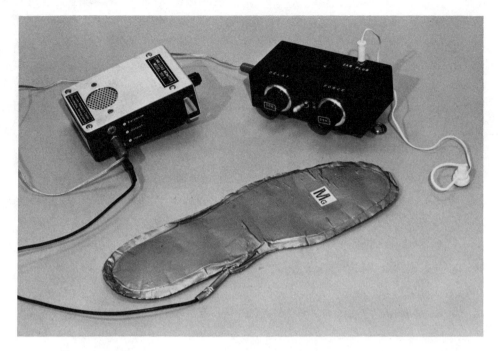

Figure 9. Components of the modified Krusen Limb Load Monitor. See
text for details.

through their limbs per unit of time, our modification provides two
controls. One is for force and the other is for time over which
that force is exerted. By regulating these two controls the clinician can shape the patients' stance phase of gait with provision of
one audio feedback for appropriate weight and duration of stance
phase.

FUTURE CONSIDERATIONS

     While the preceding sections speak to remarkable advances in
the use of biofeedback for rehabilitation medicine patients, physiological explanations for the successful interaction between patient
and modality are sorely lacking. This situation is particularly
true in attempting to comprehend how patients with central nervous
system dysfunction can improve with biofeedback applications when
previous traditional physical therapies have resulted in limited
improvement. One explanation appears to suggest that biofeedback
does not elevate the function of these patients but merely returns
this function to a level that existed when traditional therapy was
terminated. In our own clinical environment, we have investigated
this possibility. All records from our patients suggest that past

therapy was more than exemplary. There is no reason to believe that
biofeedback applications merely bring a patient to a level attained
sometime in the past during administration of more conventional rehabilitation techniques. For patients with central nervous system
deficits, Brudny et al. (1977) and Wolf (1979) have offered tentative explanations for why biofeedback might facilitate improvement
in sensory-motor integrative ability. For these patients, learning
to use limbs appropriately in a more meaningful fashion must necessi-
tate the transfer of audio and visual representations of muscle
activity to proprioceptive reappreciation of muscle length changes.
Invariably, patients forsake visual or auditory feedback in favor of
observing limb movements. This transition probably is analogous to
an internalization process wherein patients relearn appropriate
muscle lengthening and contraction to effect a purposeful movement.

To achieve this transition requires use of visual and auditory
association cortices and appropriate neural circuitry to existing
subsets of viable motor neurons within the pre-central motor cortex.
These established pathways between sensory inputs and motor output
are representative of changes in plasticity within the central nervous system. Patients capable of making these changes learn to
coordinate the intent of movement with the achievement of a task.
It would appear that those patients who fail to improve with biofeedback applications probably have a significant disruption of proprioceptive pathways. This dissociation is clinically represented
by an inability to accurately perceive passive or active joint
position.

Unfortunately, basic animal models to test these presumptions
are not available. Comprehension of mechanisms to explain the efficacy of feedback or operant conditioning paradigms designed to
improve motor coordination or movement can be speculative at best.
From a clinical perspective, tools such as computerized tomography
and cerebral blood flow measurements during biofeedback training
might provide further data concerning neural substrates linked to
this modality.

In using either EMG or positional biofeedback with neurological
patients, methodologies and procedures for demonstrating the time
course over which measurable functional gains can be obtained must
be forthcoming. Concrete data on the effect of vestibular or laby-
rinthine influences on motor learning using EMG biofeedback have yet
to be reported. On an even more elementary level, training strategies regarding the duration or magnitude of contractions have failed
to consider the predominating physiological type (tonic versus
phasic) of the target muscle. The paucity of information available
on how this modality might affect motor behavior in several diagnostic entities such as multiple sclerosis, Parkinson's disease, and
Huntington's chorea is both a testimony to the infancy of this
therapeutic tool and a challenge to the clinician.

Reference was made earlier to the use of this modality within
the context of sports medicine. Similarly, feedback to improve
motor skill may soon invade the school systems of this country.
Thus, muscle feedback has potential application not only within
rehabilitation, but also within physical education and sport. Undoubtedly, exploration into the mechanisms responsible for this form
of artificial neuromuscular training and into the more complex array
of electronic machinery will follow. For clinicians concerned with
comprehending explanations of motor control paradigms, the future
holds unlimited prospects.

DISCUSSION

PARTICIPANT: Dr. Wolf, I wonder if you would comment? Do you
have any feelings about the role that ischemia may play in the paraspinal muscles, particularly in the lower back pain?

WOLF: One of the problems with low back pain is the variety of
different causes of the pain. I think that it's really hard to
think of ischemia in terms of a significant factor in chronic back
pain patients because you would think that by that time, a year or
so following whatever the injury was, and without specific neurological findings, any ischemic response would be minimized. I think
that several of our colleagues at Emory contend that this may very
well be a major cause of back pain and the justification for lumbar-
sympathetic blocks. The argument is that if you block the lumbar-
sympathetic chain, then you temporarily denervate the sympathetic
efferents to the vasculature which supplies the paraspinal muscles.
These vessels will then dilate. The muscles will relax. As the
muscles relax, the pain receptors, either within the vessels or
within the muscles, will be less active and the person will experience less pain. The difficulty there, unfortunately, is that
there's no anatomical evidence to suggest that, on the segmental
level, injection of an anesthetic into a sympathetic ganglia will
have an effect segmentally upon that muscle. I think, other than
the use of thermography, the evidence for ischemia playing a vital
role in chronic low back pain is pretty scanty right now. The difficult problem many of us have, I think, is that in terms of neurological assessments, the very fine interarticular nerves of the
dorsal rami are very difficult to assess from a clinical analysis.
And it could very well be that it is impingement upon these very
fine nerves to joints, inter-articular joints in the vertebral
column, that contribute to pain.

PARTICIPANT: If I heard you correctly, and I think I did, you
made some comment, in the first part of your presentation, that biofeedback is effective in musculo-skeletal disorders with the quali-
fication that it might not be particularly helpful in pain disorders. And I was wondering if you could expand upon that?

WOLF: O.K. Well, I think for most people in this room it's
common knowledge that if a person is going to be in prolonged pain,
this has tremendous behavioral consequences that far outweigh at
times the organic basis for the pain. And it's very difficult to
assess improvement, physical improvement, in the presence of a
chronic pain personality. To drive home the point, we deal with a
lot of chronic pain patients for whom we've been using the modality
TENS, transcutaneous electrical nerve stimulation, to try and at
least block pain. And you look at the limitations that the patient
has before you begin the treatment, during the treatment, and after
the treatment. And let's say that the person has had a shoulder
pain following a surgery. The patient just tries to bring his arm
up and he's in excruciating pain. He's been living this way for a
year and a half and then you apply the TENS and then you ask him to
do it and he's doing this (demonstrates). And you say, "Well, are
you any better?" He says, "No, it's killing me." Yet there's
obviously something he can do, visible to you, a functional correlate that he couldn't do before. Yet his assessment of his performance is somewhat clouded or distorted by virtue of the intensity of
the pain that he's experienced. You see the difference? And there-
in lies the problem. One thing that I didn't even address, if I
could just expand for one second, is the whole issue of behavioral
interventions in chronic rehabilitation patients. And I've seen
among people in this group, within BSA or even people who do not
have a direct interest in feedback, a potential marriage here of
interests in a comprehensive approach to chronic rehabilitation
patients between physicians, allied health practitioners and, say,
psychologists . . . in the psychological assessment of a chronic
stroke or spinal cord injured patient to name but two examples.
Essentially, it deals with: can we make the home environment
accessible to the patient? Might we be able to find a job for the
patient? And are there any problems in communication between the
patient and his family or his environment? Very rarely do we ask:
how does the patient feel about himself? How does he feel about
those mysterious elements that he's going to have to deal with out
there? How does the patient feel about the obvious way in which
other people view him? And how is he gonna cope with that?
Because, you know, handicaps are something that we either tend to
ignore in passing by or to grossly exaggerate, never thinking that
chronic rehab clients happen to be human beings too, and they are
very sensitized to how people interact with them. Yet this whole
notion has been completely aborted. I mean, it hasn't even begun to
be addressed yet. Here's a golden opportunity, I think, for using a
variety of behavioral interventions within an overall comprehensive
construct that could be very effective for these poor individuals.
I don't see that happening in very many places right now.

PARTICIPANT: Dr. Wolf, would you comment upon the selection of
frequency band passes in the electromyographic instrumentation, the
selection and use of it.

WOLF: Well, there are lots of arguments about different band
pass frequencies. I'll try to make this as simple as I possibly can
for the benefit of a lot of people in this audience. If volume conduction, something that we described earlier, a superfluous pickup
of activity from some area away from the actual muscle or muscle
group you want to target, is a concern, one way of dealing with that
is to use a very narrow band pass that just looks at very specific
frequency components of the EMG signal within the pickup range of
the electrodes. Since the volume conducted activity some distance
away, like across the arm or across the leg, has some very high frequency components to it, you filter those out. That will help you
narrow in on the specific components of the signal beneath the
electrodes. Then you don't have to worry as much about the interelectrode distances. I think that's a very valid consideration.
There are a few companies that have multiple band pass alternatives
you can choose from. I think one of the difficulties is in inform-
ing people about which circumstances one would want to choose a specific band pass frequency. I don't know if that really addresses
your question. I think the important thing to keep in mind here is
these different band passes on many of these different machines
aren't just put there arbitrarily. They're there for a reason. And
one of the considerations in selecting a band pass, other than using
a notch filter to eliminate cycle interference is to relate the
interelectrode distances from the device to what your overall goal
is and hence what the filter setting should be.

PARTICIPANT: I would appreciate very much if more of the
write-ups done in relation to electromyography, as well as other
feedback work, mentioned the frequency band passes used and whether
it is peak-to-peak or RMS. Because trying to understand what I'm
doing in relation to what somebody else has done is dramatically
affected by the lack of that knowledge of the presence of it.

WOLF: That's a very good point.

PARTICIPANT: Dr. Wolf, can you speak for a moment on how you
would approach a person with spasmodic torticollis that's fairly
severe, to where it's present maybe 80-90% of the time and has to be
controlled with the limbs?

WOLF: A few of my colleagues deal with spasmodic torticollis.
We haven't seen that many patients. Every spasmodic torticollis
patient that I've seen has a psychogenic component to that problem.
If you take a very detailed history, you'll find either from the
patient or a relative or friend of the patient that there is a clear
relationship in time between the initiation of what became a very
severe torticollis and some major or unusually traumatic event in
that individual's life. We've had very little success with the
treatment of spasmodic torticollis, especially using a primary strategy of the reduction of activity in the hyperactive sternocleido-

mastoid or upper trapezius muscle, whether this has been done in terms of specific targeted training or targeted training in combination with some form of relaxation therapy. By poor results, I mean people who can demonstrate changes that could be significant, if you were to attach numbers to them, but insignificant if you were to attach time to them. Because very shortly, within a few months after treatment, they're coming back with a severe problem. Now to answer your question, I don't really know what to tell you about what to do. We haven't come up with any one treatment strategy that's very effective.

PARTICIPANT: Dr. Wolf, have you had any experience working with stammerers or stutterers? I have a a young boy who's 18, a very placid individual, but he has very severe cluttered speech and when I ask him to speak deliberately like this (enunciates slowly and clearly), he has no trouble whatever. But as soon as he starts thinking, it just blocks. I wonder if you've had any experience in the musculature of speech and training this.

WOLF: We've worked with some of our speech therapists who've had patients with articulation problems, some of them stammering, some of them just difficulty in making sounds. There are two things that are clear: one is that it's very difficult with surface electrodes to record in isolation from laryngeal muscles, as has been reported in the literature quite frequently; and two, what seems to be more effective, instead of targeting from muscles of speech or even muscles of mastication, is recording from peripheral muscles such as the upper trapezius during relaxation training and to undertake speech training in combination with reduced levels of activity from those kinds of muscles. I don't think we really know what we're doing if we try to target, unless we insert fine wires into the laryngeal muscles. Now, what hasn't been revealed in the literature, as best I can tell, is what the correlation is between electromyographic activity patterns in those muscles and speech deficits. And perhaps if that was made clear, then a qualified ENT man or someone else knowledgeable in electromyography could develop specific training strategies with in-dwelling electrodes. But I don't think we've gotten to that level of sophistication yet.

REFERENCES

Amato, A., Hersmeyer, C. A., & Kleinman, K. M. Use of electromyographic feedback to increase inhibitory control of spastic muscles. Physical Therapy, 1973, 53, 1063-1066.

Baker, M. P., Regenos, E., Wolf, S. L., & Basmajian, J. V. Developing strategies for biofeedback applications in neurologically handicapped patients. Physical Therapy, 1977, 57, 402-408.

Baker, M. P., Hudson, J. E., & Wolf, S. L. A feedback cane to
     improve the hemiplegic patient's gait. Physical
     Therapy, 1979, 59, 170-171.
Basmajian, J. V. Control and training of individual motor
     units. Science, 1963, 141, 440-441.
Basmajian, J. V. Muscles alive: Their functions revealed by
     electromyography (3rd ed.). Baltimore: Williams &
     Wilkins, 1974.
Basmajian, J. V., Kukulka, C. G., Narayan, M. G., & Takeke, K.
     Biofeedback treatment of foot-drop after stroke compared
     with standard rehabilitation technique: Effects on
     voluntary control and strength. Archives of Physical
     Medicine and Rehabilitation, 1975, 56, 231-236.
Basmajian, J. V., Regenos, E., & Baker, M. P. Rehabilitating
     stroke patients with biofeedback. Geriatrics, 1977, 32,
     85-88.
Berrol, S., Finseth, F., Yarnell, S. K., & Ralph, K. Biofeed-
     back of rectal sphincter transplant. Archives of
     Physical Medicine and Rehabilitation, 1980, 61, 468.
Binder, S. A., Moll, C. B., & Wolf, S. L. Evaluation of EMG
     biofeedback as an adjunct to therapeutic exercise in
     treating the lower extremities of hemiplegic patients.
     Physical Therapy, 1981, 61, 886-893.
Booker, H. E., Rubow, R. T., & Coleman, P. J. Simplified
     feedback in neuromuscular retraining: An automated
     approach using electromyographic signals. Archives of
     Physical and Rehabilitation, 1969, 50, 621-625
Brown, D. M., & Basmajian, J. V. Bioconverter for upper extrem-
     ity rehabilitation. American Journal of Physical
     Medicine, 1978, 57, 233-238.
Brown, D. M., Nahai, F., Wolf, S. L., & Basmajian, J. V.
     Electromyographic biofeedback in the reeducation of
     facial palsy. American Journal of Physical Medicine,
     1978, 57, 183-190.
Brown, D. M., DeBacher, G. A., & Basmajian, J. V. Feedback
     goniometers for hand rehabilitation. American Journal
     of Occupational Therapy, 1979, 33, 458-463.
Brudny, J., Korein, J., Levidow, L., Grynbaum, B. B., Lieberman,
     A., & Friedmann, L. Sensory feedback therapy as a modal-
     ity of treatment in central nervous system disorders of
     voluntary movement. Neurology, 1974 24, 925-932.
Brudny, J., Korein, J., Grynbaum, B. B., Friedmann, L. W.,
     Weinstein, S., Sachs-Frankel, G., & Belandres, P. V. EMG
     feedback therapy: review of treatment of 114 patients.
     Archives of Physical Medicine and Rehabilitation, 1976,
     57, 55-61.
Brudny, J., Korein, J., Grynbaum, B. B., & Sachs-Frankel, G.
     Sensory feedback therapy in patients with brain insult.
     Scandinavian Journal of Rehabilitation Medicine, 1977,
     9, 155-163.

Brudny, J., Korein, J., Grynbaum, B. B., Belandres, P. V., &
    Gianutsos, J. G. Helping hemiparetics to help them-
    selves. Journal of the American Medical Association,
    1979, 241, 814-820.
Coers, C., & Woolf, A. L. The innervation of muscle. A biopsy
    study. London: Oxford, 1959.
Fernando, C. K., & Basmajian, J. V. Task force report of
    Biofeedback Society of America: Biofeedback in physical
    medicine and rehabilitation. Biofeedback and Self-
    Regulation, 1978, 3, 435-455.
Finley, W. W., Niman, C. A., Standley, J., & Ender, P. Frontal
    EMG training of cerebral palsy children. Biofeedback
    and Self-Regulation, 1976, 1, 332-333.
Gianutsos, J., Eberstein, A., Krasilowsky, G., & Goodgold, J.
    EMG feedback in the rehabilitation of upper extremity
    functions: Single case studies of chronic hemiplegics.
    International Neuropsychological Society Bulletin, 1979,
    12-22.
Harrison, V. F., & Mortensen, O. A. Identification and
    voluntary control of single motor unit activity in the
    tibialis anterior muscle. Anatomical Record, 1962, 144,
    109-116.
Howson, D. C., Report on neurosuscular reeducation. Ithaca:
    ISIS Medical Instruments Inc., 1976.
Hurd, W. E., Pegram, V., & Nepomuceno, C. Comparison of actual
    and simulated EMG biofeedback in the treatment of
    hemiplegia. American Journal of Physical Medicine,
    1980, 59, 73-82.
Jacobs, A., & Felton, G. S. Visual feedback of myoelectric out-
    put to facilitate muscle relaxation in normal persons
    and patients with neck injuries. Archives of Physical
    Medicine and Rehabilitation, 1969, 50, 34.
Johnson, H. E., & Garton, W. H. Muscle reeducation in
    hemiplegia by use of electromyographic device.
    Archives of Physical Medicine and Rehabilitation, 1973,
    54, 320-322.
Jones, A. L., & Wolf, S. L. Treating chronic low back pain: EMG
    biofeedback training during dynamic movements.
    Physical Therapy, 1980, 60, 58-63.
Kelly, J. L., Baker, M., & Wolf, S. L. Procedures for targeted
    EMG biofeedback training in the hemiplegic upper extrem-
    ity. Physical Therapy, 1979 59, 1500-1507.
Kukulka, C. G., Brown, D. M., & Basmajian, J. V. A preliminary
    report: Biofeedback training for early finger joint
    mobilization. American Journal of Occupational Therapy,
    1975, 29, 469-470.
Lee, K. H., Hill, E., Johnston, R., & Smiehoeowski, T.
    Biofeedback for muscle retraining in hemiplegic
    patients. Archives of Physical Medicine and
    Rehabilitation, 1976, 57, 588.

Long, C., & Brown, M. E. Electromyographic kinesiology of the
      hand: Muscles moving the long finger. Journal of Bone
      and Joint Surgery, 1964, 46-A, 1683-1706.
Marinacci, A. A., & Horande, M. Electromyogram in neuromuscular
      reeducation. Bulletin of the Los Angeles Neurology
      Society, 1960, 25, 57-71.
Middaugh, S. J. EMG feedback as a muscle reeducation technique:
      A controlled study. Physical Therapy, 1978, 58, 15-22.
Middaugh, S. J., & Miller, M. C. Electromyographic feedback:
      Effect on voluntary muscle contractions in paretic sub-
      jects. Archives of Physical Medicine and
      Rehabilitation, 1980, 61, 24-29.
Mroczek, N., Halpern, D., & McHugh, R. Electromyographlc
      feedback and physical therapy for neuromuscular
      retraining in hemiplegia. Archives of Physical Medicine
      and Rehabilitation, 1978, 59, 258-267.
Nafpliotis, R. Electromyographic feedback to improve ankle
      dorsiflexion, wrist extension and hand grasp. Physical
      Therapy, 1976, 56, 821-825.
Owen, S. McL., Biofeedback in rehabilitation. Rehabilitation
      Gazette, 1974, 17, 46-49.
Regenos, E. M., & Wolf, S. L. Involuntary single motor unit
      discharges in spastic muscles during EMG biofeedback
      training. Archives of Physical Medicine and
      Rehabilitation, 1979, 60, 72-73.
Schneider, S., Scaer, R., Groenwald, D., & Atkinson, R. H. EMG
      techniques in neuromuscular rehabilitation with cord
      injured patients. National Paraplegia Foundation
      Newsletter, 1975, 4-10.
Seymour, R. J., & Bassler, C. R. Electromyographic biofeedback
      in the treatment of incomplete paraplegia. Physical
      Therapy, 1977, 57, 1148-1150.
Skrotzky, K., Gallenstein, J. S., & Ostering, L. R. Effects of
      electromyographic feedback training on motor control in
      spastic cerebral palsy. Physical Therapy, 1978, 58,
      547-551.
Spearing, D. L., & Poppen, R. Single case study: The use of
      feedback in the reeducation of foot dragging in a
      cerebral palsied client. Journal of Nervous and Mental
      Diseases, 1974, 159, 148-151.
Sprenger, C. K., Carlson, K., & Wessman, H. C. Application of
      electromyographic biofeedback following medial meniscec-
      tomy. Physical Therapy, 1979, 59, 167-169.
Wolf, S. L. Essential considerations in the use of EMG biofeed-
      back. Physical Therapy, 1978, 58, 25-31.
Wolf, S. L. Anatomical and physiological basis for biofeedback.
      In J. V. Basmajian (Ed.). Biofeedback: principles and
      practice for clinicians. Baltimore: Williams & Wilkins,
      1979.

Wolf, S. L. Electromyographic biofeedback in exercise programs. The Physical and Sports Medicine, 1980, 8, 61-68.

Wolf, S. L., Baker, M. P., & Kelly, J. L. EMG biofeedback in stroke: Effect of patient characteristics. Archives of Physical Medicine and Rehabilitation, 1979, 60, 96-102.

Wolf, S. L., Basmajian, J. V., Russe, C. T. C., & Kutner, M. Normative data on low back mobility and activity levels: Implications for neuromuscular reeducation. American Journal of Physical Medicine, 1979, 58, 217-229.

Wolf, S. L., & Hudson, J. E. Feedback signal based upon force and time delay: A modification of the Krusen Limb load monitor. Physical Therapy, 1980, 60, 1289-1290.

Wolf, S. L., Baker, M. P., & Kelly, J. L. EMG biofeedback in stroke: A one year follow-up on the effect of patient characteristics. Archives of Physical Medicine and Rehabilitation, 1980, 61, 351-355.

Woolridge, C., & Russell, G. Head position training with the cerebral palsied child: An application of biofeedback techniques. Archives of Physical Medicine and Rehabilitation, 1976, 57, 402-414.

BEHAVIORAL ASSESSMENT AND TREATMENT OF FECAL INCONTINENCE

Bernard T. Engel

Gerontology Research Center (Baltimore)
National Institute on Aging
National Institutes of Health, PHS
U.S. Department of Health and Human Services
Bethesda
The Baltimore City Hospital
Baltimore, MD

INTRODUCTION

Fecal incontinence is diagnosed by the presence of soiling or
staining on the clothing. Soiling means the appearance of stool;
staining means discoloration but no stool. Fecal incontinence is a
disorder which can affect individuals of any age. Milne (1976)
estimated the incidence of fecal incontinence in the general population to be 1/1000. However, it is most likely to be present in
young children or the elderly.

Incontinence can be caused by many factors; however, in most
cases there is no clear-cut cause. In children, incontinence can be
associated with congenital, neurological deficits--e.g., approximately 40% of all children who are born with spina bifida are incontinent (Lorber, 1971). However, in a series of 34 children with
fecal incontinence, Liebman (1979) could not identify any organic
cause in 95%. It also is usually the case in elderly patients that
there is no clear-cut causal event associated with the presence of
incontinence. Furthermore, in many elderly patients the disorder is
progressive with an indefinite onset--i.e., at first there are
merely occasional "accidents"--but worsening course. Although there
are no accurate data, there is general agreement that incontinence
(fecal or urinary) is the major reason why elderly patients are
placed in nursing homes. Management of incontinence seems to be a
much more serious problem than does management of confusion or other
signs of senile dementia.

In addition to congenital, neurological factors such as spina
bifida or Hirschsprung's disease, there are a number of clinical
conditions which can produce incontinence as one of its effects.
These include endocrine disorders such as hyperparathyroidism, hypo-
thyroidism or diabetes (incontinence secondary to diabetic neuro-
pathy); immunological disorders such as scleroderma; or iatrogenic
problems such as rectal surgery or chronic treatment with anticholi-
nergic drugs such as the phenothiazine compounds or the anti-
Parkinsonian drugs which sometimes are given with phenothiazines.

Incontinence can occur because of an inability of the patient
to retain stool, or it can occur in association with chronic, severe
constipation. The seeming paradox of incontinence in the face of
stool retention can be understood by a consideration of the physiology of the rectum. Stool retention results in distention of the
rectum--so-called megacolon. Distention increases the pressure
against the internal sphincter until it is no longer capable of
functioning as a barrier against the passage of stool. In addition,
the sensation of rectal fullness is mediated by stretch receptors in
the rectum. In the case of megacolon the upper limit of sensitivity
often is exceeded so that the addition of fecal matter to the
already distended colon is not sensed. It is noteworthy, however,
that during periods of severe, sustained constipation--e.g., three
or four weeks without a bowel movement--patients often report sensations of extreme fullness and discomfort. They also are reported
to become irritable as stool accumulates (Schuster, 1977).

ANATOMY AND PHYSIOLOGY OF THE ANAL SPHINCTERS

Figure 1 illustrates the normal responses of the anal sphincters to rectal distention. The normal stimulus to the sphincters is
the appearance of stool in the rectum.   However, this natural event
can be simulated by briefly inflating a balloon in the rectum, as
depicted in Figure 1. As a result of this stimulus the internal
anal sphincter relaxes and the external anal sphincter contracts.
These responses are topographically different because the internal
sphincter is a smooth muscle and is innervated by the autonomic nervous system, whereas the external anal sphincter is a striated
muscle and is innervated by the somatic nervous system (see
Schuster, 1968, for a detailed discussion of the anatomical and
physiological characteristics of these sphincters). The relaxation
response of the internal anal sphincter probably is a reflex which
is elicited by rectal distention.   However, the phasic contraction
of the external sphincter probably is a highly overlearned response
(Whitehead & Schuster, 1980; Engel, in press; Whitehead, Orr, Engel,
& Schuster, in press). Relaxation of the internal sphincter is
necessary to permit normal excretion to occur. This reflex is
absent in patients with Hirschsprung's disease. As a result, these
children retain stool and suffer from overflow incontinence. Contraction of the external anal sphincter is necessary for continence.

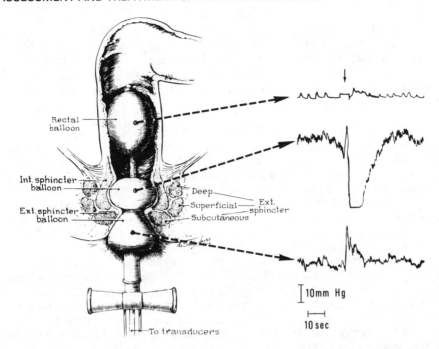

Figure 1. The normal responses of the anal sphincters to rectal distension.

The inability or unwillingness of a patient to contract this sphincter appropriately will result in incontinence of solid stool. In many such patients this skill is readily learned (or relearned), thereby rendering them continent.

DIAGNOSTIC ASSESSMENT OF INCONTINENT PATIENTS

Fecal incontinence is a psychophysiological disorder (Engel, in press). No matter what the etiology of the problem, the major consequences of the disease are social as well as medical. Furthermore, as I indicated earlier, in many cases of incontinence, particularly in children or in elderly patients, it is not possible to pinpoint a causal mechanism. In disorders of this sort, it frequently turns out to be the case that behavioral factors such as secondary gains resulting from caretaking, or psychological factors such as depression contribute significantly to the natural history of the disease. In evaluating incontinent patients, one needs to collect a number of data which are important in evaluating the patient. Table 1 is an outline of the clinical history one would obtain from a typical patient. The history might be carried out with the patient, or with a parent or guardian if necessary. The history would elicit data which would enable one to characterize the symp-

toms, especially their development and severity. The history also
would be designed to determine the role of trauma or disease in the
disorder. Finally, the history would attempt to elicit data about
the patient and the family which might be important in influencing
the outcome of therapy. Note the extent to which the clinical
history focuses on behavioral material.

The extent to which behavioral factors are important in the
evaluation of a patient is great. This suggests very strongly that
behavioral factors also will be important in influencing the outcome
of therapy. In fact, as I shall show below, for most incontinent
patients, the treatment of choice is behavioral therapy. In many
patients behavioral factors need to be assessed extensively, even
before treatment is begun. This is especially so if there is a
suggestion during the clinical interview that the patient is getting
secondary gains--e.g., attention from others in his environment--
from his symptoms. Other reasons for carrying out a behavioral analysis would be to learn whether the patient has regular toileting
habits, what the severity of the incontinence is, or what the extent
of the patient's ability to cooperate in his treatment is. Since I
have already described in some detail how one might carry out a
behavioral analysis of an incontinent patient (Engel, in press), I
will not repeat it here.

In many cases of incontinence one should carry out a rectal
manometry study (Schuster, Hookman, & Hendrix, 1965). This study
will enable one to evaluate: a) the ability of the patient to perceive stool in his rectum; b) the competence of the anal sphincters;
and c) the ability of the patient to respond appropriately to rectal
distention. Since the procedures for carrying out rectal manometry
have been described in several publications (e.g., Engel,
Nikoomanesh, & Schuster, 1974; Cerulli, Nikoomanesh, & Schuster,
1979; Whitehead, Parker, Masek et al., in press) I will not review
the techniques in detail here. The clinician who is interested in
applying the behavioral treatments described below should read these
articles carefully, since the procedures for assessing sphincteric
function differ significantly depending upon the nature of the associated pathology. Furthermore, since one uses rectal manometry to
treat incontinent patients, and since there are very important pro-
cedural differences in how one treats patients with differing etiologies, it is imperative that one have a full understanding of the
methodology before trying to apply it.

TREATMENT

Overflow Incontinence

Young (1973) has described a behavioral strategy which is used
widely to treat patients with chronic fecal retention. This method

Table 1

DIAGNOSTIC ASSESSMENT OF A PATIENT WITH FECAL INCONTINENCE

I.   Clinical history

    A.   Symptom features

        1.   Onset characteristics

        2.   Progession

        3.   Current status

        4.   Specific features

            a.   Duration

            b.   Frequency

            c.   Quality

    B.   Medical history

        1.   Injuries

        2.   Surgeries

        3.   Other illnesses

    C.   Patient characteristics

        1.   Age

        2.   Mental ability

        3.   Affective status

    D.   Family history

II. Physical examination

    A.   Structural abnormalities

    B.   Motor and sensory ability

III. Specific tests

utilizes a combination of classical conditioning, operant conditioning, and standard medical procedures. It is well known that many
subjects experience an urge to defecate within about 1/2 hour after
a meal. This is especially true in the morning. This sensation has
variously been attributed to a gastro-colic, ileocolic or gastro-
ileo-colic reflex. Whether such putative reflexes exist or whether
the sensation is learned seems clinically unimportant. The most
important point is that the patient be encouraged to toilet within
20-30 minutes after eating breakfast, and to attempt to defecate.
The toileting and in particular defecation should be accompanied by
appropriate rewards (see Young, 1973, for a strategy used with
children; Rovetto, 1979, for a strategy used with adults).

In order to optimize the behavioral strategies, at least one
principle of sound medical management needs to be met: the
patient's rectum should have adequate stool to assure that he can
have a bowel movement, but not an excessive amount of stool which is
likely to cause a reduction in sensation and/or a risk of impaction.
This principle should be met by two interventions: first, the
patient's diet should include substances which will facilitate the
formation of soft, well-formed stools; and second, the patient
should use suppositories or enemas to empty his rectum when he has
been unable to have normal bowel movements for an extended period of
time. A common practice in this procedure is to advise the patient
to use suppositories when he is unable to have a bowel movement for
two consecutive days.

Biofeedback

Biofeedback is the treatment of choice for fecal incontinence
secondary to any of several organic causes. Biofeedback has been
successfully applied in the treatment of incontinence associated
with various medical disorders such as irritable bowel syndrome,
rectal prolapse, stroke, Crohn's disease or scleroderma (Cerulli,
Nikoomanesh, & Schuster, 1979); and with incontinence associated
with various surgical procedures such as hemorrhoidectomy, laminec-
tomy, fistulectomy, prolapse repair, polypectomy, abcess drainage or
benign tumor removal (Cerulli et al., 1979). In addition, Whitehead,
Parker, Masek, Cataldo, & Freeman (in press) have shown that children with histories of spina bifida also can be treated successfully.

There are two features which make biofeedback clinically useful. First, 70 to 75% of all patients show 90% or greater improvement. Second, depending upon the age of the patient and the
underlying pathology, learning can occur within one to four training
sessions given over two or three week intervals. Furthermore, once
a patient has been successfully treated, he seems to retain the
skill indefinitely. Thus, biofeedback is extremely cost effective.

I have explained the treatment procedure in detail elsewhere (Engel, Nikoomanesh, & Schuster, 1974; Engel, 1978). Briefly, the treatment is based on the diagnostic procedure known as rectal mano-metry (Schuster, Hendrix, & Mendeloff, 1963; Schuster, Hookman, & Hendrix, 1965). In this procedure a stimulating balloon is inserted into the rectum and recording balloons are placed at the internal and external anal sphincters. Stimulation of the rectal balloon via a brief distension of the balloon results in reflex relaxation of the internal anal sphincter and voluntary contraction of the exter-nal anal sphincter (see Engel, in press). The magnitude of the sphincteric responses is directly proportional to the magnitude of rectal distension. In the normal subject one can see such responses even at very small distensions--e.g., 5 ml of air. In an incontinent patient one often can see that the patient fails to emit an appro-priate external sphincteric contraction. In most of the post-traumatic or medically ill adult patients, one can see that the threshold below which no sphincteric response is emitted is above normal, i.e., incontinence appears to be associated, _in part_, with inappropriate reactivity of the sphincter. I have italicized the phrase, _in part_, to emphasize that the defect lies partially in the performance of the sphincter. Another aspect which many of these patients share is that they often do not properly integrate the responses of the two sphincters. Thus, the external sphincter response may occur too late so that it fails to prevent stool expul-sion during the relaxation phase of the internal sphincteric reflex.

Treatment for the patients with diminished sensitivity is administered in three stages. The first stage is a routine, diag-nostic manometric study during which the threshold sensitivity of the external sphincter is determined. In the second stage, the patient is shown the manometric tracings which occur during repeated rectal stimulations in which sub-threshold or near-threshold dis-tending volumes are used. During this stage the patient is encour-aged to produce normal external sphincteric contractions which are integrated with internal sphincteric relaxations--before beginning this training, the patient is told clearly what a normal response should be. Frequently, the patient is shown Figure 1. Patients usually learn this control rapidly--i.e., within about 30 to 50 trials. Often, as the patient becomes more proficient, the dis-tending volume is decreased to improve discrimination.

The final stage of training is a series of trials during which the patient is selectively shown his response or the response is withheld. This procedure is designed to wean the patient from the gadgetry and to transfer the patient's skill to normal life situa-tions. One aspect of this training is to convince the patient that he can contract his sphincter appropriately without feedback.

Patients with spina bifida present a very different clinical problem than do the patients reviewed above. These patients typically are unable to emit an external sphincteric contraction. Instead they respond with sphincteric relaxation. In these cases, the distending volume used initially needs to be very small, and only as the patient shows an ability to contract his sphincter is the volume increased (Whitehead et al., in press). Training in these patients typically takes more sessions than does training in the adult patients cited above. However, since these patients also tend to be quite young, age plays a role in the training (see the section on motivation/reinforcement). There is one other aspect to treatment in these patients. Very often these children have never been continent, and very often neither their parents nor their physicians ever expected them to become continent. As a result, many of these children were never trained to toilet themselves. The therapist should investigate this possibility thoroughly, since it may turn out to be necessary to teach the patient how to undress and how to use a toilet.

Dietary Procedures

Prescription of diet is a usual medical approach in the treatment of various colonic or rectal disorders. However, adherence to dietary prescription is a behavioral management problem. In severe cases of non-compliance one needs to assess the determinants of non-compliance through the use of appropriate behavioral procedures (see Engel, in press). However, even in the case of a cooperative patient, the therapist should explain the function that the dietary procedure is supposed to serve. In incontinent patients, adding bulk to the diet serves the dual purposes of improving stool formation and facilitating evacuation at desired times. The therapist always should try to incorporate sound dietary practices with behavioral interventions. Occasionally, we have seen patients—especially elderly patients—who failed to respond to dietary procedures, and who showed only limited improvement following biofeedback procedures, but who showed full recovery following a combination of dietary and biofeedback modification.

Motivation/reinforcement

Motivation or reinforcement contributes to the treatment of incontinence in many kinds of patients. Foxx and Azrin (1973) have discussed these issues in detail in the treatment of mentally retarded patients and I will not deal with those patients at all. However, some problems do arise in many of the patients described above. Although the social reinforcement for continence is very strong and is almost always sufficient to maintain learning in adult patients, it may not be adequate in children. One needs to apply the principles of behavioral analysis and behavioral management (this may include parents as well as children) to assure compliance in many of these subjects. Otherwise it may turn out that the secondary gains associated either with receiving care or giving care may override the primary gain of continence. One also needs to attend to problems of reinforcement during biofeedback training in the clinic. Adult patients should be reinforced verbally--e.g., "good," "you can do better than that," etc.--after each trial early in training. However, such reinforcement should be faded as the patient shows signs of becoming more self-sufficient. Children, especially young children, respond best to material rewards such as candy or toys. It is important that these rewards be made contingent on performance.

SUMMARY

Fecal incontinence is a physical sign, not a disease. It may have very different etiologies in different patients. Thus, treatment must be adapted to fit the disorder. Behavioral procedures such as classical conditioning, operant conditioning (including biofeedback) and dietary control are very powerful means of treating incontinence. However, one must evaluate each patient appropriately, both medically and behaviorally, in order to assure rational treatment choice and optimal outcome.

DISCUSSION

PARTICIPANT: Perhaps you could refresh my memory and provide a relatively simple screening test to rule out on neurogenic deficiency of sphincter control. Generally, what I do is a simple pin-prick around S-4 and then just a digital exam gives me some idea of tonus. Anything else?

ENGEL: Yes. That's very good. If you'd ask the patient to squeeze, that would give you a notion of motor strength. You may have diminished motor strength, but potential recovery of function. Sometimes you'll have diminished motor strength simply because the patient isn't practicing anymore. Whenever possible, rectal manometry is certainly worth doing. There are a hundred or more laboratories throughout the country and certainly several in this area, in the Los Angeles area and perhaps the Bay Area as well, where rectal manometry can be done, and you can get an assessment of your patient. Where there is a dysfunction in sphincter capacity you can certainly should try biofeedback, because it is so fast, so cost effective.

PARTICIPANT: Many of my patients have fecal incontinence in association with some degree of atherosclerotic-cerebrovascular disease. And could you get a little more specific in defining where your cut-off has been in terms of mentation and ability to utilize this particular biofeedback procedure?

ENGEL: I would think that, in most of those patients, biofeedback is not indicated. I would guess that the sphincter performance

is adequate, and that the deficit there is in remembering, timing,
and motivation. And I would think their behavioral and contingency
management would be more important. I would get the patients on a
regular schedule coupled with a good diet. That will improve matters considerably. It won't cure the problem, but it will improve
matters. Because, after all, fecal incontinence, defecation, I
should say, if the stool is well formed, is only going to occur once
every day or two. So, if you can get them on a good timing schedule, you'll be well off. Many of those patients present with double
incontinence. That's a whole different problem. I might mention in
passing that Dr. Whitehead and I have established, in the National
Institute on Aging, a geriatric continence clinic. We're very
interested in researching the problems of both fecal and urinary
incontinence in the elderly. We're seeing patients 65 and older.
I'll give you a clinical vignette with one patient which might be
useful. We saw an 80-year-old woman who'd been referred to us by
her private physician because she was incontinent even though he had
put her on a good bran diet and Metamucil. We used biofeedback with
her because she had a reduced sensitivity in her sphincteric
responses. We judged that even though she had improved her ability
to sense rectal distension, she would probably not have sufficient
muscle strength to respond. The coupling of diet with biofeedback
training was sufficient. This lady's been continent now for close
to a year. If you use a rational approach, you can get some very
gratifying results. Returning to your problem, I think you have to
treat it as a behavioral management problem.

PARTICIPANT: How sophisticated does the patient have to be to
know that biofeedback can be effective, somebody with some mild
chronic learning syndrome who also has a sphincter impairment?

ENGEL: Oh, no that's not a major problem. We've taught six-
year-old spina bifida children.

PARTICIPANT: I've always been fascinated at the speed with
which this training is accomplished and I wonder if you could comment on the implications of that, for learning theory perhaps, in
general, or just for training of visceral function? I mean you've
got people here who've had a problem for 20 years, and in 20 minutes
we're beginning to see very rapid functional change.

ENGEL: Let's get some perspective on this. That's a little
dramatic. There have been problems for several years, but whether
20 years, is a bit much. First of all, when I said that the
learning occurred between 1-4 sessions, I was talking about the
adult incontinent patients. In the case of the spina bifida
children it takes 4-6 sessions. (laughter) Well, but it takes
longer and he's asking about learning theory. It's gratifying that
it goes so fast but still in terms of theory, there is an acquisition, there is a development. In a session, which is about two

hours or so, we do stimulate the rectum about 50 times so there are a lot of trials. Then we tell the patient to go home and practice, squeeze several times throughout the day to strengthen muscles. So there is a lot of practice outside. But the training in the clinic, in adult incontinent patients, comes very, very quickly. It's an extremely highly over-learned response, and unless you've had significant cerebral damage, they don't forget how to do something even though they may have lost the motor capability.

PARTICIPANT: Have you done any work with paraplegic or quadri-plegic patients with spinal cord section?

ENGEL: No.

PARTICIPANT: Is there any work being done at all? Do you know? Say there is some cord connection left, but by and large the patient is essentially without any control.

ENGEL: I don't know of any work specifically with fecal, with rectal sphincteric control. We have been successful in training paretic patients, and Whitehead has been successful in training spina bifida children. However, I know of no work with patients who have had complete transections of the cord.

REFERENCES

Cerulli, M. A., Nikoomanesh, P., & Schuster, M. M. Progress in biofeedback conditioning for fecal incontinence. Gastroenterology, 1979, 76, 742-746.

Engel, B. T. Fecal incontinence and encopresis: A physiological analysis. In R. and W. Whitehead (Eds.) Psychophysiology of the Gastrointestinal Tract: Experimental and Clinical Aspects. New York: Plenum, in press.

Engel, B. T. The treatment of fecal incontinence by operant conditioning. Automedica, 1978, 2, 101-108.

Engel, B. T., Nikoomanesh, P., & Schuster, M. M. Operant conditioning of rectosphincteric responses in the treatment of fecal incontinence. New England Journal of Medicine, 1974, 290, 646-649.

Foxx, R. M., & Azrin, M. H. Toilet Training in the Retarded. Champaign, Illinois: Research Press, 1973.

Liebman, W. M. Disorders of defecation in children. Postgraduate Medicine, 1979, 66(2), 105-110.

Lorber, J. Results of treatment of meningomyelocele: An analysis of 524 unselected cases, with special reference to possible selection of treatment. Developmental Medicine and Childhood Neurology, 1971, 13, 279-303.

Milne, J. S. Prevalence of incontinence in the elderly groups. In
    E. L. Willington (Ed.), Incontinence in the Elderly. London:
    Academic Press, 1976.
Rovetto, F. Treatment of chronic constipation by classical
    conditioning techniques. Journal of Behavioral Therapy and
    Experimental Psychiatry, 1979, 10, 143-146.
Schuster, M. M. Motor action of rectum and anal sphincter in
    continence and defecation. In C. F. Code (Ed.), Handbook of
    phystology Section 6, Alimentary Canal. Vol. IV, Motility.
    Washington, D.C.: American Physiological Society, 1968,
    2121-2146.
Schuster, M. M., Hendrix, T. R., & Mendeloff, A. T. The internal
    anal sphincter response: Manometric studies on its normal
    physiology, neural pathways, and alteration in bowel disorders.
    Journal of Clinical Investigation, 1963, 42, 196-207.
Schuster, M. M., Hookman, P., & Hendrix, T. R. Simultaneous
    manometric recording of internal and external anal sphincteric
    reflexes. Bulletin of Johns Hopkins Hospital, 1965, 116, 79-88.
Whitehead, W. E., Orr, W. C., Engel, B. T., & Schuster, M. M.
    External anal sphincter response to rectal distension: learned
    response or reflex. Psychophysiology, in press.
Whitehead, W. E., Parker, L. H., Masek, B. J., Cataldo, M. F., &
    Freeman, J. M. Biofeedback treatment of fecal incontinence in
    meningomyelocele. Developmental Medicine and Child Neurology,
    in press.
Whitehead, W. E., & Schuster, M. M. Therapeutic application of
    biofeedback in digestive disorders. In J. E. Berk (Ed.),
    Developments in Digestive Diseases. Philadelphia: Lea and
    Febiger, 1980.
Young, G. C. The treatment of childhood encopresis by conditioned
    gastroileal reflex training. Behavioral Research and Therapy,
    1973, 11, 499-503.

BIOFEEDBACK THERAPY WITH CHILDREN

Judith A. Green

Biofeedback and Stress Management Group
Boulder, Colorado
Psychotherapy and Biofeedback Associates
Greeley, Colorado

Children are not immune to stress and stress related illnesses.
Psychosomatic disease, behavior disorders, and exacerbation of
learning disabilities and organic disease such as epilepsy and diabetes may all be stress related in children. This paper describes
the use of biofeedback training and adjunctive techniques in the
treatment of these disorders in children, in a clinical setting.
The treatment goal is psychophysiological self-regulation through
relaxation and stress management, self-image, and cognitive change.

In a diversified private practice, data on the treatment of
specific disorders accumulate slowly and do not illustrate the variety of methods used in clinical applications. I will focus therefore on general principles of biofeedback therapy and on the details
of the therapeutic procedures which I use in working with children.

PRINCIPLES OF BIOFEEDBACK TRAINING AND SELF-REGULATION

Principles of Learning. Self-regulation of physiological processes through biofeedback training is based upon principles which
are common to all learning. Consider the events which occur in
learning to throw darts. The intention to throw the dart and hit
the target leads to the act of throwing; the player observes the
position of the dart and thus receives information feedback on the
accuracy of the throw. With the use of this information four processes may occur: 1) the player changes behavior and throws again,
receiving new information; 2) the player becomes increasingly aware
of his own actions; 3) control of body actions and mental set and
thus control of the dart is achieved; and finally 4) the actions

involved in hitting the bulls-eye become habitual and the player no
longer consciously produces each movement.

Learning self-regulation through biofeedback training is similar except that the information which is "fed back" to the trainee
is information about a physiological process such as heart rate,
hand temperature (blood flow), muscle tension (EMG), or brainwaves
(EEG), which the trainee is learning to control. It would be difficult, perhaps impossible, to learn to hit the bulls-eye while blindfolded, simply because there would be no information feedback with
which the player could judge the last throw and thus adapt the next.
It is equally difficult to regulate consciously bodily processes
without information feedback. With the use of sensitive biofeedback
instruments, however, physiological processes are amplified and con-
verted into meaningful signals which inform the trainee of ongoing
changes in the process being monitored. The trainee uses the continuous feedback of information to make changes in the desired
direction.

Rationale. That all learning is based on information fed back
is clear. But how does the introduction of information enable the
individual to make changes in normally involuntary processes? The
same question can be asked of the voluntary system--how can the
intention to act lead to the action? Interestingly, even in the
voluntary nervous system, the link between afferent and efferent
pathways does not reach consciousness. We have no direct conscious
awareness of neuronal events in the central nervous system, and yet
exquisite control is possible.

Figure 1 (Green & Green, 1977) diagrams the steps involved in
the regulation of conscious and involuntary processes through biofeedback training. Stimuli which reach consciousness through sensory perception of external events, such as the ringing of a fire
alarm, Box A, and their conscious and unconscious emotion/mental
repercussions, Box B, and ideations, volitions, and emotions internally generated by the individual, Box B and Box H, have unconscious
neurologial ramifications, Box C. The crucial element for self-
regulation of physiological processes is Line 2, the connection between emotional/mental responses and limbic system responses.
Studies which demonstrate this link have been necessarily crude, as
are the responses generated in laboratory situations via limbic stimulation and ablation, compared with the seemingly infinite elaboration of emotional/mental responses in humans. Nonetheless, it seems
certain that the limbic system plays a unique role in the dialogue
between emotional/mental states and physiological processes, particularly autonomic "involuntary" processes. The translation of
emotional/mental responses into physiological responses occurs via
the extensive neuronal connections between amygdala and other limbic
structures, hypothalamus, and reticular formation (Isaacson, 1974;
Livingston & Escobar, 1971). When a biofeedback instrument is

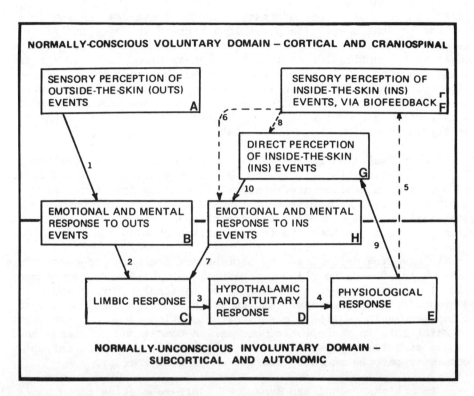

Figure 1. The steps involved in the regulation of conscious and involuntary processes through biofeedback training. (From Beyond Biofeedback by Elmer and Alyce Green. Copyright 1977 by Delacorte Press/Seymour Lawrence. Reprinted by permission of the authors and the publisher.)

introduced into the system of emotional-mental response/physiological response, the normally unconscious physiological response is brought into the conscious domain. This is indicated in Box F of the diagram. The trainee now perceives the response, Box G, and has an immediate emotional/mental and behavioral reaction to it. This reaction in turn stimulates limbic system responses, Line 3. The feedback instrument responds to the change with new information, which the trainee perceives. Again, emotional/mental and behavioral responses occur as the trainee uses information to create the desired change. The trainee becomes increasingly more aware of internal processes and finally gains physiological control.

Thus, a cybernetic loop is established which incorporates mental/emotional and physiological responses, and simultaneously, conscious and unconscious responses. Biofeedback is described as a technique which brings mind and body together simply because it is a

reflection of both. The information feedback mirrors the physiology, and to some degree the physiology mirrors the emotional/mental
state. When working with physiological processes which are highly
sensitive to emotional/mental input, such as blood flow and electrodermal response (EDR), the trainee very quickly sees the relationship between emotions and ideations and physiological responsivity.
The extent to which the trainee regulates emotional/mental responses
is reflected in a degree of limbic system regulation, and consequently in physiological self-regulation.

The crucial link in the stress response and in the development
of psychosomatic illness seems to be the connection of limbic system
and emotional/mental events, whether originating from external or
internal stimuli. The same link is used to promote psychophysiological health through biofeedback training and therapeutic techniques
which promote a pro-homeostatic interaction of mind and body.

Intervening variables. As biofeedback training progressed from
research laboratory to clinic, important variables were recognized
which intervene between the external or internal stimulus and
emotional/mental responses: attitudes, beliefs, and expectations.
It has become increasingly clear that the client's mental set plays
a crucial role in therapeutic outcome. A commitment to change and
a sense of self-responsibility for one's health are essential to
successful outcome and are promoted as part of therapy.

Educational model and homework. Self-regulation through
biofeedback training, as the term implies, is a learned skill
requiring good instruction, and in most cases, consistent practice.
Consequently, homework exercises are an integral part of biofeedback
therapy. The burden of change, which takes time and effort, is on
the client. These ingredients make biofeedback a unique form of
therapy which follows an educational model of change.

Physiology of stress and relaxation. Consideration of the
physiology of stress and relaxation is important in understanding
the use and effectiveness of biofeedback training in the treatment
of psychosomatic disorders. While the neurophysiology of the stress
"fight-or-flight" response has been extensively studied, its neurophysiological counterpart, relaxation, was given little attention in
medicine and physiological research until the last decade. Relaxation is not merely the absence of stress. Relaxation seems to be an
"active" principle which brings the body back to healthy homeostasis. Consequently, relaxation is a major component of biofeedback
therapy in the treatment of many disorders. It is the pervasive physiological effect of relaxation which accounts for its broad application and effectiveness, just as the pervasive physiological effect
of stress accounts for its extensive role in illness.

In summary, biofeedback training and adjunctive techniques in

the treatment of psychosomatic illness, use relaxation to create
prohomeostatic physiological change, feedback of information to
increase awareness and control, with emphasis on positive expecta-
tion, learning and self-responsibility, and the powerful interaction
of body and mind.

INTRODUCING THE CHILD TO BIOFEEDBACK TRAINING

Children are referred to biofeedback training by physicians,
teachers or parents. Often both child and parents are uncertain of
the uses and methods of biofeedback. To insure understanding by all
family members and to prevent the child from being singled out as
"the sick one," I invite the entire family to the first session.
This also gives me an opportunity to observe family interaction, an
important variable in the child's illness and behavior.

I introduce myself as a biofeedback teacher. I explain that I
teach ideas and skills, I like to be asked questions and like to ask
questions. The use of questioning as a method of teaching is a
valuable tool which assures me that the child and family understand
biofeedback training. In addition, I "set up" questions so that the
child will have correct answers, which provides numerous positive
"ah-ha" experiences and guarantees the child's attention. This
approach also reinforces the educational goal of biofeedback therapy
and supports a crucial element in successful outcome, self-responsibility, with its helpmates, practice and persistence. Most children
are eager to gain this type of self-responsibility, and thus
biofeedback training has an inherent appeal.

I introduce biofeedback training and the underlying principles
through seven basic ideas. In brief, these ideas and accompanying
questions flow in this manner:

IDEA #1
MIND-BODY
TEAM

> We have a mind-body team that works together all the
> time. Does everyone in this room have a body? Does
> everyone in this room have a mind? Give me some
> examples of when your mind and body work together. What
> about when you are sleeping?

IDEA #2
STRESS
RESPONSE

> Naturally, we want to train the whole team, so in

biofeedback training we work with the body and the
mind. Now we need to talk about stress and what it does
to the body. What does it mean when we say "I feel
nervous or uptight?" Tell me about a time when you were
stressed or uptight. What did your body do when you
felt like that? Yes, mind and body react to stress in
certain ways. Tell me how your mind feels when you are
stressed. And how does your body feel?

IDEA #3
YOUR
SYMPTOM

Your (headache) is like a stress response. This is how
it works (the physiology of the symptom is simply
described when appropriate). Remember all the things
your body does when you feel stressed? Well, your blood
flow also changes. When you are scared or

IDEA #4
BLOOD FLOW
AND STRESS

nervous, even just a little, blood flows away from your
hands and feet. Where do you think it goes? Why
would blood do that? Yes, the body does this to help
us. Remember we called this the fight-or-flight
response. If blood flows away from your hands when you
are uptight, do you think they get warmer or colder?
Now what do you think happens to the blood when you

IDEA #5
RELAXATION

relax? And do your hands get colder or warmer? When do
they get warmer? And what happens to your blood flow
when you relax? If you wanted to teach people how to
relax, what would you teach them to do? Yes, and here
is a biofeedback machine that helps you to learn to
relax, and you will have this machine to use at home.
What else happens inside your body when you relax? If
you have been running and you relax, what happens? What
if you are scared and you relax? And what happens to
your mind when you are relaxing? If you are scared and
you relax, what happens to your mind? What do you think
would happen if you were sick and you really relaxed?
Yes, relaxation changes your body. When you relax you

really change your own body, and of course your mind
too. You can see that relaxation is pretty powerful,
and that is why a lot of our work in biofeedback is
learning how to relax.

IDEA #6
INFORMATION
FEEDBACK
AND
LEARNING

Now we have two more ideas before we use the biofeedback
machine. We need to talk about how we learn, how we
learn anything at all. Imagine that you are learning to
play darts for the first time. What do you do? And,
you see where the dart lands and that tells you
something. We call this information feedback. What do
you do with this information? Yes, and you try again,
and you get more information. Do you think you could
learn to hit the bulls-eye blindfolded? Why not? So we
need information to learn. Now what do you think the
word "biofeedback" means? Yes, and what can you do with
the information from your body? Yes, you can learn to
control your body. Of course, since your mind and body
work together all the time you also learn to control
your mind. Now here is the last idea. Do any of you
play an instrument or have any of you learned a sport?
What do you do over and over so that you will get better
and better? Right, you practice.

IDEA #7
PRACTICE,
NEW HABITS

You practice and practice until your new skill becomes
a ____? Now this is also true of learning relaxation
and learning to control your mind and body. You practice until the new skill becomes a habit. We can think
of your body as having a bad habit. But you can teach
it a new and better habit. Biofeedback, like other
tools we will use, takes practice. And as you know, if
you have a bad habit, say in playing the piano, it takes
time to undo it and learn the right thing. That is true
of mind habits too. If you have the habit of getting
angry or scared, it takes time to learn new mind habits,
but you can.

At this point, I demonstrate the portable temperature feedback

unit for use at home and have the client read through the homework
record sheet and the autogenic phrases (Figures 2 and 3) which are
the basis of home practice. If the child is too young to read, the
parents will help with the homework. Older children train themselves and keep their own records.

Training begins with a primary relaxation exercise: deep, even
breathing. After one of the children has demonstrated breathing to
the group, each family member attaches the thermistor of a temperature feedback unit to the middle finger of the dominant hand. I
point out that trying too hard to relax doesn't work because the
body just gets stressed. This is an important concept for successful training. In the first session I read the phrases, pausing
after each phrase while it is repeated silently by the children.
Children are very good at raising finger temperature, often better
than parents, and are instantly rewarded with success. If the temperature drops, the child can usually relate this to feeling
nervous. In either case, the link of body and mind and the effects
of relaxation or stress have been demonstrated. The first session
ends with a brief review of the basic ideas and homework plans.

Clinical sessions with children usually include review of
homework, five minutes of hand temperature training, EMG feedback,
imagery, and sharing. When appropriate, the child brings school
work to the session.   In working with children who have behavior

MY NAME __J__ DATE 1-23-80 DAY Wed.
I PRACTICED FOR _____ MINUTES. I PUT THE THERMISTER ON: RIGHT HAND _____
                                                         LEFT HAND ✔
MY TEMPERATURE STARTED AT 79.1 AND THE HIGHEST SCORE WAS 96.3
TO HELP MYSELF RELAX I USED: (SLOW DEEP BREATHING) (RELAXATION PHRASES)
    THE BODY SCAN   IMAGERY   MY TAPE   AND _____
TO HELP MY MIND AND BODY WORK TOGETHER I USED MY IMAGERY OF clouds
    MY MOTTO   MY SPECIAL PHRASE   AND _____
DURING THIS PRACTICE MY BODY FELT: VERY RELAXED (SOME RELAXED) NOT RELAXED
DURING THIS PRACTICE MY MIND FELT: VERY RELAXED (SOME RELAXED) NOT RELAXED
AFTER THIS PRACTICE I WILL FEEL: (VERY RELAXED) SOME RELAXED NOT RELAXED
MY IMAGERY WAS: CLEAR AND STRONG   SOMEWHAT CLEAR AND STRONG   WEAK
TODAY I FELT: WONDERFUL SAD GOOD HEALTHY HAPPY MAD (GLAD) ANGRY
    DUMB SILLY SMART (SICK) SUPER LOVING MEAN KIND RELAXED
RIGHT NOW I FEEL: WONDERFUL SAD GOOD HEALTHY HAPPY MAD GLAD
    ANGRY HURT DUMB SILLY SMART (SICK) SUPER LOVING MEAN
    KIND RELAXED
I REMEMBERED TO TURN OFF THE BIOFEEDBACK MACHINE   YES ✔
I WILL USE MY MOTTO, IMAGERY AND RELAXATION BEFORE FALLING ASLEEP ✔

Figure 2. Homework sheet.

```
                    RELAXATION AND IMAGERY PHRASES FOR _____

   I FEEL QUITE QUIET
   I AM BEGINNING TO FEEL QUITE RELAXED
   MY FEET FEEL HEAVY AND RELAXED
   MY ANKLES, MY KNEES, AND MY HIPS FEEL HEAVY, RELAXED AND COMFORTABLE
   MY TUMMY AND THE WHOLE MIDDLE PART OF MY BODY FEEL RELAXED AND CALM
   MY HANDS, MY ARMS, AND MY SHOULDERS, FEEL HEAVY, RELAXED AND COMFORTABLE
   MY NECK, MY JAWS AND MY FOREHEAD FEEL RELAXED.  THEY FEEL COMFORTABLE AND SMOOTH
   MY WHOLE BODY FEELS CALM, HEAVY, COMFORTABLE AND RELAXED
   MY WHOLE BODY IS RELAXED AND MY HANDS ARE WARM, RELAXED AND WARM
   WARMTH AND HEAVINESS ARE FLOWING INTO MY HANDS, THEY ARE HEAVY AND WARM
   I CAN FEEL THE WARMTH AND HEAVINESS FLOWING DOWN MY ARMS INTO MY HANDS
   I AM A LIMP RAG DOLL WITH HEAVY ARMS AND LEGS AND A SMILE ON MY FACE
   I AM A LIMP RAG DOLL WITH HEAVY ARMS AND LEGS, AND MY MIND IS CALM AND PEACEFUL
   MY WHOLE BODY IS RELAXED, RELAXED, RELAXED AND MY HANDS ARE WARM, WARM, WARM
   I AM RELAXED AND CHEERFUL AND FULL OF LIFE


   MY OWN PHRASE:_____
```

Figure 3. The autogenic phrases which are the basis of home practice.

problems, except hyperactivity, I may use techniques such as role playing and imagery more than biofeedback training.

BIOFEEDBACK TRAINING AND ADJUNCTIVE TECHNIQUES

Biofeedback training: Hand temperature and EMG feedback instruments are the primary biofeedback tools which I use with children. All children are given portable temperature feedback units for home practice (Electromedics, BF100) and are expected to practice daily. Children are surprisingly consistent in keeping training and symptom records when the records are designed for easy scoring.

EMG Feedback training begins with forearm electrode placements and a game of "guess your tension." By squeezing his or her hand, the child creates tension which registers on the feedback meter at some level, i.e., ten microvolts. When this level is easily held and regained after relaxation, all feedback is removed. The child is instructed to tighten again and guess when the tension is at ten microvolts exactly. Without feedback, this is initially a difficult task. Guessing trials are alternated with feedback trials. The child is coached to "feel what ten feels like" in fingers and arm. Typically, after six to eight trials the child is fairly accurate in estimating "ten" without feedback. The point: the body is a good

biofeedback machine when we pay attention to it; we can learn to
feel without a machine.

For basic relaxation and training in self-regulation, forehead
EMG feedback is used. A time-period integrator is helpful for
keeping minute-by-minute scores which can be graphed and easily compared to provide a motivation for beating the last score. In hand
temperature and EMG training, children win prizes for improving
scores; the child picks a prize from a bag of toys and games.
Ninety five degrees Fahrenheit is the training goal for a prize,
often first achieved in home training.

I use electrodermal response (EDR) feedback to demonstrate the
power of emotions on the body through a game in which I try to guess
a secret number that the child has chosen, based on the EDR. I have
not used EDR feedback as a relaxation tool.

Adjunctive Techniques: Biofeedback training used in isolation without adjunctive techniques or cognitive support, as in some research
paradigms, may be a relatively weak tool. Studies employing biofeedback in this condition demonstrate its least effect, sometimes
impressive nonetheless. When biofeedback is used in conjunction
with adjunctive techniques, which interact synergistically, biofeedback becomes a more powerful tool. When adjunctive techniques are
used, however, as in clinical practice, the relative contribution of
biofeedback training cannot be assessed. This situation may be
perplexing to clinicians but cannot be avoided when maximum clinical
effect is sought.

The use of adjunctive techniques naturally varies with the
client, and in some cases biofeedback training itself is the adjunctive technique. The techniques described here are the major tools
which I use with biofeedback training.

Breathing. Chronic poor breathing habits appear to be associated with poor health and stress reactions in children and adults.
When deep even breathing is established, clients report significantly enhanced relaxation and the ability to increase peripheral
blood flow. Often deep breathing is the most effective "at the
scene of the crime" stress management technique. In general,
children are good breathers, although the breath may be shallow or
held during problem solving and stress. Occasionally, breathing is
reversed, pulling in the abdomen with the inbreath, and pushing out
with the outbreath. Breathing exercises are particularly important
for asthmatic children, practiced when the airways are open and used
when wheezing. Children are instructed to watch their breathing
throughout the day and note when and how it changes.

Breathing instruction begins with the child on the floor, one
hand on the chest, one on the abdomen. The child breathes as usual,

noticing how the hands move. In relaxed breathing, the lower hand
should move while the chest hand is essentially quiet. A larger
breath begins with the abdomen, and the chest follows with ribs
expanding. The instruction to breathe into the lower hand and imagine filling the lungs like balloons is usually sufficient to establish correct breathing. Basic breathing exercises include slowing
and extending the breath, deep even breathing, even counting of the
inbreath and outbreath, pausing at the end of the outbreath, progressive rapid breathing, and breathing out tension or anger. All
relaxation exercises begin with deep even breathing.

   Body scan. The body scan is a body awareness exercise. It
begins, "with the power of your mind, put your attention into the
bottoms of your feet. Really feel the bottoms of your feet and nod
your head when you can really feel how the bottoms of your feet
feel. Now your ankles, really feel how your ankles feel," and progresses to the top of the head, pausing to allow verbal feedback at
stomach, shoulders, and hands. The child is instructed to stop at
any part of the body that feels tense or uncomfortable and just
"breathe out" through that part, feeling the tension floating away.
If a particular part of the body is being worked with, such as the
lungs, we pause there to feel that part and bring warmth and relaxation to it. The body scan is concluded by spreading the attention
from top of the head to bottoms of the feet and giving the whole
body and mind a word of thanks for doing so well. Progressive
relaxation, or alternately tensing and relaxing muscle groups
(Jacobson, 1957), is a good precurser to this exercise.

   Limp rag doll. This is a simple exercise in which the child
pretends to be a limp rag doll. I pick up the child's arms and legs
and feel how floppy they are, no bones, no muscles, just like a limp
rag doll. The heaviness of the limb with relaxation is easily
experienced, especially when I let go. Interestingly, when I used
this exercise with a group of learning disabled children, six of the
eleven children were surprised to discover their arms still hanging
in the air after I let go. Apparently these children had little
proprioceptive feedback from their bodies. I have wondered if these
were the six hyperactive children in the class.

   Imagery. I introduce imagery by talking about juicy sour
lemons, vinegar pickles, and black spiders crawling up your arm.
The point is easily made—images have power. Imagery is therefore a
useful tool for inducing physiological change as well as psychological change. I began using imagery with children because fantasy is
a child's forte, and I now use imagery with all clients.

   The use of imagery varies with the needs of the client. Basic
imagery techniques include imagery for enhancing relaxation; inspection and a clean-up tour of the body area in need, such as the
lungs; healing the body; desensitization; dialogue; self-image

change; and stress rehearsal.

Imagery exercises begin with relaxation. I explain the importance of relaxation with a simple analogy: if all the kids in the
classroom are out of their seats and making a racket, no one hears
when the teacher speaks. But if everyone is seated and paying
attention, everyone hears when the teacher speaks. Your body is the
classroom and your mind is the teacher, so it is important to have
the body quiet before talking to it with imagery. The reverse is
true also, the teacher needs to be quiet and pay attention in order
to hear the kids, so it is important to quiet the mind as well so
that it will hear when the body speaks.

Brief relaxation exercises and colored dots. Learning brief
relaxation techniques and using these techniques throughout the day
is an important aspect of training. Brief relaxation practiced many
times a day enhances healthy homeostasis and relaxation as a natural
state, increases awareness of tension, and prevents a buildup of
tension in the body. Short relaxation exercises for children
include deep breathing, being a limp rag doll, head and shoulder
rolls, and a self-directing phrase. Brief imagery can also be
incorporated into these short exercises. The child is given bright
colored stick-on dots to place around the house and school books as
reminders to use the short exercises.

Cognitive techniques. Teaching, coaching, and sharing are
important in biofeedback therapy. In an unusual case, an asthmatic
child grew molds which we examined with a microscope, discovering
that molds are "quite beautiful and interesting, and certainly harmless looking." I use biology books and other materials when appropriate. Kaufman (1976) has written and illustrated an excellent
book on human anatomy and physiology for children.

"Self-talk" is another cognitive tool which enhances self-
awareness and change. Self-talk refers to the internal monologue
with which we often occupy our minds. Children are instructed to
watch their self-talk, noticing what kinds of messages they are
giving to themselves. Negative messages are changed into positive
messages.

Children also create "mottos" and special phrases which rein-
force positive self-image, self-direction and symptom reduction: "I
read relaxed," or "when I wake I'll be breathing perfectly." Dis-
identification is used: "I have asthma but I'm not my asthma," "I
have anger but I'm not my anger." Assessment and cultivation of
positive beliefs, attitudes, and expectations are continual throughout therapy. Occasionally, I use the Children's Personality
Questionnaire (1975) as an interview to stimulate communication and
to facilitate assessment of the child's mental set.

Tapes. Relaxation and imagery cassette tapes for home practice are commonly used in biofeedback therapy, particularly when home practice trainers are not available. I rarely use tapes as the primary home training tool. Often, however, after several clinic sessions the child and I make a tape of favorite relaxation phrases, breathing exercises, motto, and imagery. The tape is made specifically for the child's needs and goals.

Several creative tape sets for relaxation and self-management are commercially available for school or clinic use (Lowenstein, 1976; Lupin et al., 1976; Stroebel, 1980).

To test the child's ability to relax under stress, I created a "stress practice tape" which presents numerous verbal, writing, and reading tasks through a barrage of distraction stimuli. Children watch finger temperature feedback while using the practice tape as an indication of how well they can relax when stressed.

Biofeedback game. The Biofeedback Game is another test of relaxation skill while stressed. This game (The Biofeedback Game, Humedics Corp.) is designed for two players, or for playing one hand against the other. I play with the child and I am a good challenger. The game gives auditory feedback and bounces a luminated "red ball" toward the goal of the player with the most rapidly increasing hand temperature or decreasing EDR; when the goal is reached, a number is added to the player's score. Games of this type and feedback instruments which run trains and helicopters in relation to change in a physiological variable may hasten training and symptom reduction in children. When the flight of a helicopter is dependent upon relaxation, the hyperactive child is confronted with a serious dilemma, but has a powerful incentive to learn to quiet body responses and curb "stimulus-bound" behavior.

CLINICAL EXAMPLES

Migraine headache. J. was referred to biofeedback training by her neurologist with a diagnosis of migraine headache. Her medications were periactin, amitriptyline, Tylenol, and aspirin. She reported continual right sided headache with associated vomiting during the previous four months and was out of school much of that time. J. appeared to be shy and unassertive and spoke in a high, soft voice, in contrast to her mother, the verbal boss of the family. Nonetheless, J. became conversant in the first session and very pleased to have her own machine and be in charge of her training. J. kept good headache and home practice records, and was diligent in practice. Figure 4 shows headache data. In the third week of training, she began attending school part time and by the end of training was in school full time again. Figure 2 is an example of J.'s homework sheets.

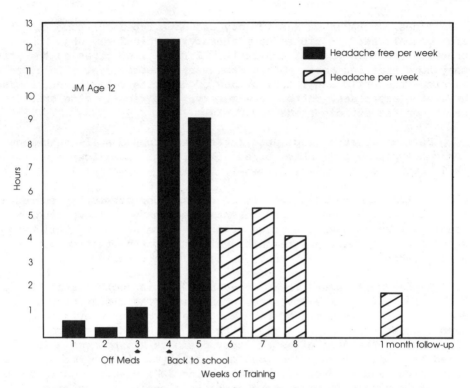

Figure 4. J's headache data.

J. began biofeedback training with cold hands. In the first
session, her finger temperature dropped from 76.1 degrees Fahrenheit
to 75.8 degrees Fahrenheit. Training at home was better, with
scores up to 91.8 degrees Fahrenheit in the first week. After four
weeks of training, J. could easily increase hand temperature in the
clinic, and was successfully reducing or eliminating headaches.

In general, children have low forehead EMG scores, but J. produced
8 to 6 microvolts peak-to-peak, Biofeedback Systems, PE-3. After
two sessions she was able to reduce tension somewhat.

J. put colored dots around her room and in school notebooks as
reminders to practice the short relaxation exercises throughout the
day. She also used a Biotic Band (Bio-Temp Products, Inc.) at
school and at home after returning the biofeedback machine at
termination.

In the one-month follow-up phone conversation, J. reported that
she was essentially headache-free. She continued to practice daily
and was happy to report that she could turn off headaches at will.
J. is unusual in the duration of her headaches and degree of vaso-

constriction. To her advantage were a keen desire to eliminate
headaches and an appreciation of the mind-body team.   Midway
through training, she asked if it were possible to get rid of a wart
with the mind. A visualization was created and by the time of her
follow-up report the wart on her hand was gone.

Hyperactivity. K. was referred to biofeedback training by his
learning disabilities teacher. She described him as hyperactive
with an IQ of 79, but with qualities which convinced her that he had
more potential than he was demonstrating in school. After five
weeks training, K. was given the WISC in the children's training
room during the Thanksgiving vacation. Overall I.Q. was 102, with
performance of 114. K. was 10 years old but was functioning at
second grade level. He was taking 30 mg. of ritalin on school days.

K. appeared to be unusually short, thin, and undernourished.
The only sign of hyperactivity was the rapid movement of his eyes as
he took in all the details of my office. His parents were poorly
educated, used punishment as the main form of discipline, and were
open about their dislike for the child. The dynamic of family reinforced hyperactivity was clear; the only way to get attention was to
"act out," even if this meant punishment.

A correlary of this dynamic (and supported by the family myth
that K. was hyperactive and retarded because at age two he consumed
a bottle of baby aspirin) was a "destined-to-fail" attitude which he
maintained. For K., failure was much safer than success. He predicted his own failure in tasks, and he often ripped holes in his
school papers and destroyed his work.

K. came to the clinic twice during the school week and on
Sundays. Sunday was used for biofeedback training and tutoring
while K. was off ritalin for the weekend. On this day he was
trained by a supportive male intern at The Menninger Foundation,
where this work was conducted. K. demonstrated rapid mastery of
hand temperature training, and after four sessions, EMG training
began. A feedback myograph, BFT 401C, was used for auditory and
visual feedback; the unit was attached to a Time Period Integrator,
BFT 215C, which provided minute averages of EMG level (RMS) measured
from forehead electrode placement. I recorded minute scores, and
usually started the time period myself; the goal was 10 minutes,
which took as long as 60 minutes in the beginning of training. At
the end of training, K. worked for two-minute periods, and easily
trained for 20 minutes in much shorter sessions. Scores were
charted on a large graph on the training room wall. At the 20 unit
level a purple line was drawn across the chart, the "surprise line."
K. knew that if he could keep his scores below the surprise line for
ten consecutive minutes, he would receive a wonderful surprise.
When he reached this goal, the line was lowered to the ten unit
level. Figure 5 shows means and standard deviations of EMG scores
over sessions.

EMG training brought out K.'s hyperactivity. The initial
sessions were mainly wiggle feedback and scores were kept high by an
unconscious facial grimace. A mirror was used for feedback of the
grimace and the habit subsided in three weeks. During scored
minutes, I often repeated autogenic training phrases and gave continual reinforcement. K. was instructed to use his own phrases
silently; his favorite personal phrase which he created was "my hair
is smooth." Periodically, during a no-count minute, K. was asked to
wiggle and grimace as much as possible to see how high a score he
could get. This helped to enhance his awareness of tension and
relaxation.

Two highlights of training are noteworthy. In session 12, K.
spontaneously said "You go and type, I'll do this myself." The
equipment, time period start button, and scoring pad were placed on
a board across the arms of the recliner in which K. worked. He
trained alone for six exciting minutes and then took off the electrodes and dashed to my office with his scores. He was thrilled by
his achievement and shared his scores with the entire staff.
Session 13 was also solo, and K. trained for ten minutes. These
self-mastery sessions appear to be a breakthrough in training, as
seen in Figure 5. Previously, the high means and standard deviations were due to K.'s tendency to sabotage a low score by wiggling
in the next minute, unable to maintain success. Only session 9 dif-

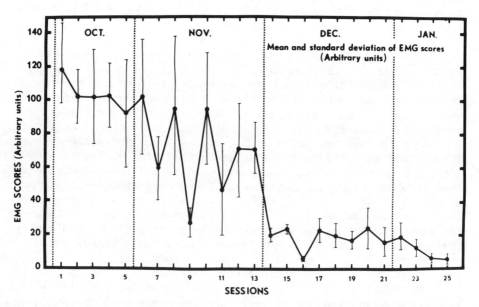

Figure 5. The means and standard deviations of K.'s EMG scores over
sessions.

fered from this pattern, but on that day K. had a stomach ache.

The second highlight of training concerns session 16. In session 15, I informed K. that on the day of the next session, if he kept his scores below the surprise line, he would get a very special surprise, which happened only on that day. K. immediately replied "I can't." At the beginning of session 16, however, he remarked "I think I can," and minute after minute remained absolutely still. Again, K. shared his victory with the staff, going from office to office receiving hugs. K. had grown from a shy, destined-to-fail child to one who could accept a challenge and enjoy his success. K. won his second prize in the 25th session, and with that success we concluded EMG training.

K. continued therapy through April. During that time we focused on academic tutoring and withdrawal from medication. At the end of the school year, K. was on 15 mg. ritalin daily and did not use the medication in the following year.

I visit the classroom when working with children. During four classroom visits, I was surprised to find that K. was not particu- larly hyperactive in school as verified by his teacher on the Conners Teacher Rating scale (Conners, 1969) which she scored weekly. In fact, K. alternated between periods of mild hyperactivity and disorganized work and prolonged periods of "staring into space." The Conners Rating Scale on hyperactivity showed little change except brief increases with each 5 mg. reductions in ritalin. Predictably, two scales which did change were leadership and assertiveness. K.'s teacher kept a small weather thermometer in her desk for K. to use when he felt himself becoming "hyper." Occasion- ally he assigned himself to the "time-out" box and relaxed.

I believe that in this case hyperactivity had no organic basis, but was a behavioral problem stemming from environmental sup- port of "acting out" behavior and poor self-image. Biofeedback training was valuable primarily as a tool for helping K. gain self- mastery and experience success, which in turn facilitated the devel- opment of a positive self-image.

Asthma. E. was referred to biofeedback training by her pediatrician. She was ten years old and developed asthma in the first month of life. She was allergic to pollens, molds, dust, ani- mal hair and feathers. E.'s regular medications were Alupent, Slophyllin, and weekly allergy shots; she used an inhalant, and received adrenalin shots as needed. Medication dosages were changed many times during training, increasing or decreasing according to E.'s condition. E. was an adopted child and held some anger toward her parents and younger siblings, feeling that she alone would have been enough. She also carried on a continual struggle with her mother over medication use, with mother feeling caught between daughter and allergist.

E. was a very bright and verbal child, easily understanding the purpose of the training. Her specific goals were to reduce medication, to be able to play harder and longer with no wheezing, and to "stop asthma." She was able to apply relaxation and breathing techniques to reduce wheezing under most conditions if she stopped her activities and focused on relaxing and opening the lungs. On one occasion, she came to the clinic in considerable distress and was able to stop wheezing completely in fifteen minutes.

Every session with E. included hand temperature and forehead EMG feedback training, breathing, and imagery. With asthmatic clients, imagery is introduced in the first session with slow, deep breathing. After studying an enlarged diagram of a section of lung tissue, the child is instructed to visualize relaxed bronchiole muscles with air sacs expanding perfectly while practicing the breathing exercise. This training of the "mind-body team" becomes part of the homework.

E.'s home training included relaxation with the temperature feedback unit, imagery specific to her goals, measurement of peak flow before and after relaxation using a Mini-Wright Peak Flow Meter, and repetition of her special phrase before falling asleep.

When E. demonstrated sufficient relaxation skills, desensitization was initiated. Her first goal was to eliminate the feather allergy. Desensitization began with relaxation and imagery, practiced only when she was breathing perfectly. The imagery was as follows: "you are sitting in my office in the big brown chair. Tell me when you are in the chair. Notice how perfectly you are breathing. Now I come into the office with a baby quail in my hands. (Quail were readily available from an ethology research project.) I hand you the baby bird. You notice how perfectly you are breathing and you say to yourself 'A feather is just a feather. Now you cuddle the bird against your cheek, and you say to your body, 'a feather is just a feather.' You notice how easily you are breathing while you talk to the little bird and cuddle it. Now you hand the bird to me and I take it back to the nursery. You continue to breathe perfectly." This scene was rehearsed several times before E. informed me that she was ready to try out the imagery. Following relaxation, we enacted the imagery as rehearsed with one exception--there was only one bird in the quail room on that day and it had just hatched. The bird was covered with yellow down rather than beautiful feathers as baby quail are. With some trepidation, I took the bird to my office and we carried out the imagery, yellow down escaping between our fingers. Nonetheless, E. experienced no effects from this experiment. She then graduated to a feather pillow, again with no allergic reaction.

E. also wanted to work on the mold allergy and her first task
was to grow molds. She brought in a colorful piece of cheese and I
contributed a loaf of very moldy bread which we examined under the
microscope. The bread was placed in a cabinet in the training room,
and it is noteworthy that none of the asthmatic children reacted to
the mold, including one client who entered training after a severe
reaction following a school biology experiment with molds. Theoretically, relaxation in the presence of the allergen counteracted
the reaction of the immune system.

Imagery for mold desensitization was a guided fantasy. E.
visualized herself in a meadow teaming with particles of pollen,
mold, and dust which she breathed in and out as "harmless parts of
nature." She explored the woods near the meadow and discovered a
grove of large molds and green spores on the forest floor. After
examining the molds, she found a stream in which to rinse her hands,
all the time noticing how perfectly she was breathing. At the
conclusion of the imagery, she exclaimed "I was wondering how I was
going to get that stuff off!"

During one year of therapy there were a variety of setbacks and
gains, with gradual improvement in E.'s ability to increase physical
exercise and exposure to allergens without wheezing. A severe reaction during a trip to the mountains put her on a short course of
prednisone, but prior to this she had a much reduced reaction while
horseback riding. A significant change occurred when E.'s mother
gave her total responsibility for her medications. E. recorded
medication use, but whether she took it or not was up to her. With
this freedom, E. developed a sensible plan for reducing medications
based on reduced frequency of wheezing. Near the end of training,
E. broke her jaw in a car accident. The wiring of the jaws prevented her from taking her usual medications. She had no reaction
to this reduction and gradually withdrew from all medications.

At one year following termination, E. was symptom-free and
wanted her own quail. Because all baby quails look alike, she had a
difficult decision. She stood in the hot quail room for many
minutes handling the birds in search of the right one. She had no
reaction to this unusual exposure.

This case was successful; not all are. Other asthmatic
children were able to stop moderate wheezing but were not able to
eliminate all medications or prevent occasional attacks. All
children made progress in reducing allergic reactions and reaction
to exercise, but not under all conditions.

These cases illustrate the use of biofeedback therapy with
three distinct disorders. In each case the focus of treatment,
duration, and outcome vary. Treatment of migraine headache is
short-term and daily home training in peripheral vasodilation (hand

warming) and adjunctive relaxation is perhaps the essential ingredient.

On the other hand, clinic sessions may be the essential ingredient in the treatment of hyperactivity, as in the case presented. Success in self-regulation via EMG feedback coupled with continual support and reinforcement produces significant self-image change, the major therapeutic outcome. In this treatment, then, biofeedback training is a vehicle for inducing positive behavioral and psychological change by providing the experience of success. I refer to this aspect of biofeedback training as "a set-up to succeed." It is difficult for a child to fail at biofeedback training. Through progressive but easily achieved goals, reinforcement, coaching, and shaping of behavior, success can be engineered. For children who often experience failure, success in biofeedback training may be a significant life change.

The long-term treatment of a serious, chronic disorder, asthma, reflects in this case the tenacity of the immune system, and may reflect psychological variables resulting from chronic illness from infancy. Nonetheless, two important results occurred in the first few weeks of training with the asthmatic children with whom I have worked--ability to reduce wheezing and counteract the fear of an attack. The knowledge "I can do something" was of inestimable benefit to these children, and is a benefit of biofeedback therapy with all children. The mental set and the ability to actually "do something" automatically facilitates return to homeostasis, and are important elements in all applications. For this reason, all my clients use a temperature feedback unit for home practice, regardless of complaint. The experience of daily success in self-regulation is a powerful catalyst for growth.

SELECTED OVERVIEW OF BIOFEEDBACK AND SELF-MANAGEMENT APPLICATIONS

To date, publications on the clinical applications of biofeedback therapy with children in private practice are scarce. Yet undoubtedly many clinicians use biofeedback therapy in the treatment of childhood disorders with positive outcome. In addition to the treatment of headache, hyperactivity, and asthma, my own work includes single cases of chronic vomiting, performance anxiety and sweaty palms, insomnia, nose bleeds, and temper tantrums, all with good results.

Limited data indicate that tension and migraine headache in children may yield more quickly to biofeedback training than other disorders, and more quickly than in adults, averaging 6-10 sessions (Werder, 1978). In an early report by Diamond (1976), biofeedback training was considered the treatment of choice for children with migraine headache.

A recent report (Olness, McParland, & Piper, 1980) describes successful results in the treatment of children with fecal incontinence using anal spincter feedback.

Several reports are available on biofeedback training and other relaxation and behavioral management techniques for treatment of asthma, reviewed by Knapp (1979) and Olton and Noonbert (1980). In general, these studies demonstrate a definite relationship between relaxation and improved bronchial functioning. In the treatment of asthma, as in other medical applications, biofeedback training and similar techniques appear to interact positively with medications, often enabling reduction or elimination of medication.

Limited but promising data indicate that children with epilepsy (Sterman, MacDonald, & Stone, 1974; Kay, Shively, & Kilkenny, 1978), and cerebral palsy (Finley, Niman, Standley, & Wansley, 1977; Kalb, 1978; Halpren et al., 1970; Wooldridge & Russell, 1976) can be helped with biofeedback techniques.

In contrast to clinical applications, reports on the use of biofeedback training and other relaxation procedures with learning and emotionally disabled children, including hyperactive children, are numerous. The majority are research studies in school settings and focus on a variety of behaviors including handwriting (Carter & Synolds, 1974; Hughes, 1979), inappropriate behavior (Walton, 1979), subvocalization (Parsky), intellectual functioning (Braud, 1978), learning disabilities (Hunter, Russell, Russell, & Zimmerman, 1976; Murphy, Darwin, & Murphy, 1977; Russell & Carter, 1978), stuttering (Hanna, 1975), and self-injurious behavior (Schroeder, Peterson, & Solomon, 1977). Several of the studies on hyperactivity have been reviewed by Bhatara (1979). Lubar and Shouse (1976) report preliminary results using sensorimotor brainwave rhythm feedback with hyperactivity; this research is still in progress.

A pilot program (Project Reptile, 1979) uses biofeedback and relaxation training and affective education with children identified as mildly to moderately emotionally handicapped. The program was designed to help teachers and students cope with daily setbacks in a positive, planned way. This program, in progress, appears to be achieving these goals.

These studies and programs indicate that children with learning and emotional difficulties in special education programs can benefit from relaxation and self-management training.

Biofeedback training and other relaxation and self-awareness techniques used in the normal classroom may be thought of as preventive medicine and are an excellent addition to the child's education. In several innovative programs, children and adolescents learn to identify stressors and stress responses and to counter stress with

relaxation. Students are given the opportunity to practice relaxation in the classroom and are encouraged to generalize this response
to other situations. An exemplary program is described by
Englehardt (1978).

CONCLUSION

Biofeedback therapy with children is a multi-faceted tool with
diverse applications. Using a combination of biofeedback training
and adjunctive techniques, children learn to alleviate symptoms
through psychophysiological self-regulation and through relaxation,
which enhances healthy homeostasis. As an aid to relaxation and
self-awareness, biofeedback therapy helps the child develop skills
for coping with stress and for counteracting the stress component in
illness, learning and emotional disabilities, and life changes. At
the same time, by virtue of its unique methodology employing self
training as its modus operandi, biofeedback therapy promotes self-
responsibility, success, and development of positive self-image,
therapeutic results which are of particular value to children with
learning, emotional, or organic handicaps.

Biofeedback therapy with children is a natural. Most children
seek self-responsibility and are eager to learn. Most children have
not yet developed a mental set of helplessness and hopelessness.
Preventing the development of illness and stress as a life style,
through intervention at an early age, is both propitious and
possible.

REFERENCES

Bhatara, V., Arnold, L. E., Lorance, T., & Gupta, D. Muscle
    relaxation therapy in hyperactivity: Is it effective? Journal
    of Learning Disabilities, 1979, 12(3), 182-186.
Bruad, C. W. The effects of frontal EMG biofeedback and progressive
    relaxation upon hyperactivity and its behavioral concomitants.
    Biofeedback and Self-Regulation, 1978, 3, 69-89.
Carter, J. L., & Synolds, D. Effects of relaxation training upon
    handwriting quality. Journal of Learning Disabilities, 1974, 7,
    236-239.
Children's Personality Questionnaire, Form A(1975), Institute for
    Personality and Ability Testing, Champaign, Illinois.
Conners, K. C. A teacher rating scale for use in drug studies with
    children. American Journal of Psychiatry, 1969, 126, 152-156.
Diamond, S. Biofeedback; choice of treatment in childhood migraine.
    Biofeedback and Self-Regulation, 1976, 1, 349.
Englehardt, L. Awareness and relaxation through biofeedback in
    public schools. Biofeedback and Self-Regulation, 1978, 3, 195.

Finley, W. W., Nieman, C. A., Stanley, J., & Wansley, K. A. Electro-
    physiologic behavior modification of frontal EMG in cerebral
    palsy children. Biofeedback and Self-Regulation, 1977, 2,
    59-79.
Green, E., & Green, A. Beyond biofeedback. New York: Delacorte
    Press/Seymour Lawrence, 1977.
Halpern D., Kottke, F. J., Furrill, C., Fiterman, C., Popp, U., &
    Palmer, S. Training of control of head posture in children
    with cerebral palsy. Developmental Medicine and Child
    Neurology, 1970, 12, 290-305.
Hanna, R. et al. A biofeedback treatment for stuttering. Journal
    of Speech and Hearing Disorders, 1975, 40, 270-273.
Hughes, H. et al. Treatment of handwriting problems utilizing EMG
    biofeedback training. Perceptual and Motor Skills, 1979, 48,
    603-606.
Hunter, S. H., Russell, H. L., Russell, E. O., & Zimmerman, R. L.
    Control of fingertip temperature increases via biofeedback in
    learning disabled and normal children. Perceptual and Motor
    Skills, 1976, 43, 3, 743-755.
Isaacson, R. L. The limbic system. New York: Plenum Press, 1974.
Jacobson, E. You must relax. New York: McGraw-Hill, 1977.
Kaufman, J. How we are born, how we grow, how our bodies work, how
    we learn. New York: Golden Press, 1976.
Kay, J., Shively, M., & Kilkenny, J. Training of sensorimotor/
    rhythm in developmentally disabled children through EEG
    biofeedback. Biofeedback and Self-Regulation, 1978, 3,
    197-198.
Knapp, T. J., & Wells, L. A. Behavior therapy for asthma: A review.
    Behavior Research and Therapy, 1978, 16, 103-115.
Kolb, B. The effects of biofeedback relaxation training on speech
    and writing skills of cerebral palsy children and adolescents.
    Dissertation Abstracts International, 1978, 38 (12-B), 6218.
Livingston, K. E., & Escobar, A. Anatomical biofeedback of the lim-
    bic system concept. Archives of Neurology, 1971, 24, 17-21.
Lowenstein, J. Relaxation tapes for children. The consciousness
    Living Foundation, Manhattan, Kansas.
Lubar, J. F. & Shouse, M. N. EEG and behavioral changes in a
    hyperactive child concurrent with training of the sensorimotor
    rhythm (SMR): A preliminary report. Biofeedback and Self-
    Regulation, 1976, 1, 293-306.
Lupin, M., Braud, L. W., Braud, W. & Duer, W. Children, parents, and
    relaxation tapes. Academic Therapy, 1976, 7, 105-113.
Murphy, P. M., Darwin, Jr., & Murphy, D. A. EEG feedback training
    for cerebral dysfunction. Paper presented at the Biofeedback
    Society of America Annual Meeting, Orlando, Florida, February,
    1977.
Olness, K., McParland, F. A., & Piper, J. Biofeedback: A new modal-
    ity in the management of children with fecal soiling. Journal
    of Pediatrics, 1980, (March), 96, 505.

Olton, D., & Noonberg, A. R. Biofeedback: Clinical applications in
    behavioral medicine. New York: Prentice Hall, Inc. 1980.
Parsky, L. M. Biofeedback induced suppression of subvocalization in
    sixth grade learning disabled children. University Microfilms,
    Box 1864, Ann Arbor, Michigan, 48106.
Project Reptile; an experience in relaxation training, biofeedback
    training and affective education for children. Porter County
    Special Education Cooperative, Emotionally Handicapped Project,
    Porter County, Indiana.
Russell, H. L., & Carter, J. L. Biofeedback training with children:
    consultation, questions, application, and alternatives.
    Journal of Clinical Child Psychology, 1978, 7, 2.
Schroeder, S. K., Peterson, C. R., Solomon, L. J., & Artley, J. J.
    EMG feedback and the contingent restraint of self-injurious
    behavior among the severely retarded; two case illustrations.
    Behavior Therapy, 1977, 8, 738-741.
Sterman, M. B., MacDonald, L. R., & Stone, R. K. Biofeedback
    training of the sensori-motor EEG rhythm in man. Epilepsia,
    1974, 15, 395-416.
Stroebel, E., Stroebel, C., & Holland, M. Kiddie QR: A choice for
    children. QR Institute, Wethersfield, Connecticut.
Walton, W. T. The use of a relaxation curriculum and biofeedback
    training in the classroom to reduce inappropriate behavior of
    emotional handicapped children. Behavior Disorders, 1979, 5,
    10-18.
Werder, D. S. An explorative study of childhood migraine using ther-
    mal biofeedback as a treatment alternative. Biofeedback and
    Self-regulation, 1978, 3, 242-243.
Wooldridge, C. P., & Russell, G. Head position training with the
    cerebral palsy child: An application of biofeedback
    techniques. Milbank Memorial Fund Quarterly, 1976, 57, 407-14.

ACKNOWLEDGEMENTS:

Special thanks to Robert Shellenberger, Ph.D., and the staff of the
Voluntary Controls Program, The Menninger Foundation, Topeka,
Kansas.

BIOFEEDBACK AND DERMATOLOGY

Robert M. Miller

Assistant Clinical Professor
U.C.L.A. School of Medicine
Canoga Park, California

The skin is the largest organ system in the body. It contains
several structures which are innervated by the autonomic nervous
system (ANS). The sympathetic nervous system (SNS) is the branch of
the ANS which seems to predominate in the skin. The structures so
innervated are the epidermal appendages, i.e., the eccrine sweat
glands, hair follicles (arrector pili muscle), and probably the
myoepithelial cell of apocrine sweat glands, and the blood vessels
of the dermia.

The eccrine sweat glands function over most of the body as an
evaporative cooling mechanism. They are, therefore, heat sensitive
and respond via heat receptors located in the hypothalamus to increases in skin and body temperatures. They may also respond via
reflexes at the level of the spinal cord. The eccrine sweat glands
on the palms and soles, however, do not function (primarily) as part
of the cooling system. They respond to emotional stimuli. From a
teleologic point of view, we can see how sweaty palms might have
afforded a better grip on a tree branch for our primate ancestors as
they fled in fear from predators. During moments of anxiety sweaty
palms are very familiar to most of us.

The chemical transmitter of the SNS is usually norepinephrine.
The chemical for the nerves supplying the sweat glands is acetyl-
choline. It is not clearly known why this is different.

The hair follicle ties into the autonomic nervous system via
the arrector pili muscles. These are smooth muscles originating in
the dermis and inserting into the hair follicles. They attach below
the sebaceous gland on the side of the follicle which forms an

145

obtuse angle with the epidermis. When the muscle contracts, the
follicle is pulled and the obtuse angle decreases, approaching a
right angle. The hair then stands up on the skin. For lower ani-
mals such as cats this might allow them to appear larger and more
ferocious. In human beings the result is "goose bumps." Lindsley
and Sassman (1938) reported on a man who could voluntarily erect the
hairs on his body.

In response to stimulation via sympathetic fibers, the blood
vessels of the dermis actively constrict, leading to a blanching of
the skin. Blushing results from vasodilation. In skeletal muscle,
vasodilation actively occurs via sympathetic cholinergic fibers. In
the skin, a cholinergic vasodilation mechanism also is present.
However, it is not clear to what extent it is due to kinins released
by sweat glands, and to what extent to actual vasodilation fibers.
Apparently both occur. Neuronally controlled vasoactivity may originate centrally or may result from an axon reflex starting in the
skin (Champion, 1970). The temperature of the skin also varies as a
function of its blood flow. In Raynaud's phenomenon, the skin becomes white and cold as the vessels constrict. If the constriction
lasts for a long time, infarction of the skin can occur. When the
vessels dilate the skin becomes red and warm. The facial blush of
embarrassment is psychogenically induced vasodilation.

In humans, the function and innervation of the apocrine glands
is poorly understood. Apocrine sweating occurs in the axilla and
auditory meatus in response to fear and evoked pain. Adrenergic
stimuli activate glands, but it is not clear whether it is by circulating adrenaline or by adrenergic nerves. The breast is a modified apocrine gland and the myoepithelial cells there are autonomi-
cally controlled.

The main, if not total, innervation of the epidermis is sensory. Whether there are autonomic fibers going to it, their function is poorly understood. The skin also has certain electrical
properties. It can conduct or resist an externally applied electrical current. The conduction of the current can be modified by emotional stimulation. An intact autonomic nervous system is necessary
for this to occur. The response to an externally applied current is
called the galvanic skin response (GSR). In 1890, Tarchanoff found
that a difference of potential could develop between two electrodes
from the skin, even in the absence of an externally applied current.
This too was modifiable by emotional stimuli. Edelberg (1967)
states the electrodermal reflex may be regarded as an increase in
the total permeability of a selective cutaneous membrane in response
to the arrival of an impulse carried by cholinergic sympathetic
nerves. The eccrine sweat gland seems to be the main site for this,
but a cellular layer, presumably in the epidermis, may also be
involved.

Knowing where the autonomic nerves go in the skin and the function of the various skin structures, we are in a better position to
discuss biofeedback for skin disorders.

As already mentioned, Raynaud's phenomenon is a disorder
characterized by marked vasoconstriction of acral structures such as
hands and feet. There are several causes such as Carpal Tunnel
Syndrome, scleroderma, etc. Coldness is usually the stimulus for
the vasoconstrictive response. The coldness can be climactic, such
as wintry weather, or local, such as removing a cold beer from a
refrigerator. Emotional stimuli may also precipitate the response.
The thrust of therapy has generally been to avoid cold stimuli.
This includes wearing gloves in cool weather and when removing objects from the refrigerator. Also, vasodilating drugs have been
used and sympathectomies have been done to eliminate the vasoconstriction.

Biofeedback has probably been tried more times for Raynaud's
phenomenon and disease than for any other skin disorder, and the
responses greatly vary. The method most commonly used is to feed
back skin temperature and to attempt to raise that temperature. It
is reported that many patients have been able to raise skin temperature 10°F. Although skin temperature has a high degree of correlation to vascular dilation and constriction, it would seem more
beneficial to be able to measure and feed back vascular activity
directly (Jacobson et al., 1978; Sappington et al., 1979; Taub &
Stroebel, 1978; Adair & Theobold, 1978).

Bird and Colborne (1980) used biofeedback to raise the skin
temperature of a 22-year-old man who had sustained a severe burn of
his flexor wrist. With training, he was able to raise his skin temperature 21°F. It was felt that his clinical improvement accelerated after the biofeedback was started.

Hyperhidrosis is a disorder characterized by excessive and prolonged eccrine sweating, usually of the palms, soles, and axillae.
It is generally considered to be emotionally induced. Local anti-
perspirants have been used with variable success. Systematic anti-
cholinergic drugs have been used, but the side effects are often
more incapacitating than the hyperhidrosis. Rickles describes a
case of a 16-year-old Caucasian male who was trained to control his
hyperhidrosis. An instrument which measured vapor pressure was used
as the sensing device. Koldys and Meyer (1979) report similar
results.

Eczema is a descriptive pattern. It is usually red and pruritic and might or might not ooze. One of the major microscopic
characteristics is intercellular edema from the epidermis. There
are a variety of causes for eczema. One is almost purely emotional.
This eczema is called neurodermatitis. Contact dermatitis is

an eczema of an allergic basis. It is a delayed hypersensitivity characterized by T (thymus stimulated) lymphocytes. Any emotionally induced component of eczema is either secondary or operant by systems we have very little knowledge of today. Often the term eczema, when used by itself, refers to atopic eczema. This is a complex hereditary disease characterized by derangements of both immediate and delayed hypersensitivity. There are increased levels of IgE and apparently depression of some components of delayed hypersensitivity. There seems to be a very strong emotional component which gives atopic eczema its other name, generalized neurodermatitis. It is part of the disease complex referred to as atopy or the atopic diathesis. It consists of allergic rhinitis, asthma, and sometimes hives. The clinical picture will evolve depending on whether the nasopharyngeal mucous membranes, the respiratory mucosa, or the skin are involved. Any of these organ systems can be involved.

Biofeedback has been used to treat atopic eczema. However, components of the eczema were not used as the information to feedback. In the study by Haynes et al. (1979), frontalis electromyographic feedback was employed. The major thrust was to decrease itching and to effect a general relaxation to decrease the emotional tone of the patients. The results were variable, but encouraging. Unfortunately, atopic eczema follows a very variable course, and normative data is hard to collect. Further work in this area needs to be done.

Dyshidrotic eczema is probably a form of atopic eczema which primarily involves the sides of the fingers and palmar surfaces of the hands. It may also involve the feet. Usually many small vesicles are seen, but the eczema can be dry. The severity varies tremendously from a few mildly pruritic vesicles to hands which are so eczematized that serum literally drips out. Hyperhidrosis is a very common finding. Because of this, dyshidrotic eczema was originally believed to be a disorder of sweat glands. Hence the name dyshidrotic eczema. Hyperhidrosis, however, is not always present and is not necessary for the diagnosis to be made. An emotional component is often clearly present. The biologic tendency to atopy is almost always found. Miller and Coger (1979) asked two questions. First, if there is a significant emotional component to dyshidrotic eczema, how does the stimulus for eczema get from the brain to the hands? Is there a humoral substance carried by the blood, or does it travel via the autonomic nervous system? Second, if it is carried by the ANS, can we alter the response with biofeedback?

Again normative data is difficult to obtain. They did, however, design the study as a double blind. Skin conductance was used as the variable to be fed back. It was chosen because it is affected by hydration of the skin and by sweat. Eczema is charac-

terized by increased hydration of the epidermis (intra- and intercellular edema). Dyshidrotic eczema often has the added feature of
hyperhidrosis.

An inexpensive instrument which measures skin conductance was
given to each patient. Normally the instruments emit a tone whose
frequency is directly proportional to the skin conductance. Half of
the instruments were reversed so the tone actually decreased as skin
conductance increased. All of the patients were instructed to
decrease the tone so as to decrease skin conductance. There were
statistically significant differences between the two groups. The
group trained to decrease skin conductance showed clinical improvement more often than the controls who were trained in the opposite
direction. They also showed a significant decrease in measured conductance and anxiety. The controls showed increased anxiety and no
significant changes in skin conductance levels.

Clearly, more research needs to be done on the effects of
biofeedback on those diseases already studied. Biofeedback might
also be used to help uncover some of the mechanisms of those
diseases. There obviously is a lot of room for speculation as to
the use of biofeedback in other skin conditions. In fact, one can
only speculate, because there is a terrible dearth of literature on
the subject.

Psoriasis is a disease characterized microscopically by epidermal changes consisting of accelerated growth rate and regular
elongation of the rete ridges. In the dermis, there is a tortuosity
and dilation of the superficial blood vessels. Clinically, one sees
redness of the psorittic plaque. The etiology is unknown. Little
more is known about the pathophysiology, especially as to what happens first. There are many treatments directed at various aspects
of the pathophysiology. One of these is the use of topical cor-
ticosteriods. These powerful drugs have many actions, one of which
is vasoconstriction. Obviously, it is not a very great leap to ask
if biofeedback could be used to constrict the dilated vessels of the
papillary dermis. If it worked, not only would biofeedback become a
useful therapeutic tool for psoriasis, but it might also shed light
on the pathophysiology of this disease.

Uriticaria has a multiplicity of causes. They range from
allergies to mast cell tumors to psychogenic causes. The final
pathophysiologic event is the same. The blood vessels dilate and
leak fluid into the dermis. This causes a swelling visible from
the surface as a welt or hive. An obvious question is, can biofeedback be used to reduce hives? Can one learn to vasoconstrict small
blood vessels and prevent the leakage of fluid?

There are a great many dermatologic diseases which are immunologic in nature. Some are mediated by immunoglobulins and some by

T lymphocytes. Examples are, respectively, Lupus erythematosus, pemphigus, and pemhigoid for immunoglobulin mediated diseases, and contact dermatitis and alopecia areata for T lymphocyte mediated disease. As Schleifer has reported, the immunologic defenses can be altered by emotional stress. Men grieving for the loss of recently deceased wives showed lower immunologic responses (Schleifer, 1980). Whether one is able to learn to alter immunologic responses, and whether biofeedback can be a method of such learning, will remain a question for a while.

We have seen how biofeedback has been used to control skin temperature, sweating, eczema, and itching. We have speculated on its use in other skin diseases. We have asked how it can be used as a therapeutic modality and as a research tool to delineate pathophysiologic mechanisms. The time has come for more people to use biofeedback on the skin, the most accessible organ of the body.

DISCUSSION

PARTICIPANT: Could I make a comment? I'd like to correct an impression you may have given regarding the use of the Radio Shack GSR. We've been through this many times over the years in biofeedback. That instrument is not suitable for clinical work, primarily because it passes too much current through the skin. If you measure the current, it's well into the milli-amp range. My research has shown you shouldn't exceed 15 micro-amps if you want to have a useful GSR. That large amount of current passed through the skin produces polarization very rapidly. Five minutes is about the longest time you can use a simple instrument like that. After that, a massive artifact gives the impression that the GSR response is reducing when in fact it's not doing that at all. There's no comparison between an instrument that is cheap and the more sophisticated, good GSRs that are on the market presently.

MILLER: Yeah, I didn't want to give that impression. But unfortunately, at the time, we were stuck with using that, finances being what they were, and we hoped to try and overcome that to a certain extent by reversing the machines, but you're right. It's not the best instrument to be used and we did this . . . we had no other choice. We went ahead with this study the way it was in the hope that if we did get some kind of positive results, then further work with more sophisticated instruments could be used. And hopefully some of you will use them. At the present time, we are just not doing work in that field any more, so we're not going to be able to do it.

PARTICIPANT: In the area of application of biofeedback in dermatitis or dermatological conditions, I think where one can look for many hints, for people in fact to practice autonomic self-regulation techniques for skin disorders and other disorders as well as immunal illnesses, it would be the autogenic training literature. If you go to Volume Two, you'll see there's a large section where people have essentially taught patients autonomic self-regulation skills to reverse pathology and, in fact, coolness is often indicated for hives, for many of the other dermatological conditions. I think that literature really would be helpful.

MILLER: Thank you.

PARTICIPANT: Some of the work that I see being done in the clinic for psoriasis, within the psychogenic framework, would be hand temperature warming, relaxation, and autogenics that Erik was talking about. In the psoriasis you're talking about swollen blood vessels and in hand warming we are talking about an increase of blood flow. Is this a contradiction? How do we look at those two factors: a psychogenic factor and a physiological factor?

MILLER: With regards to what? To urticaria, to psoriasis or what?

PARTICIPANT: Well, psoriasis, in particular, but I would . . . I'm not clear on exactly the other physiological variables in skin diseases, but I would think that the contradiction or paradox may exist in other areas too besides psoriasis.

MILLER: I'm not sure exactly what your question is, but I don't want to imply that psoriasis is strictly a psychogenic disease or that it has a simple mechanism of vasodilatation. That's only one component of it. There are a lot of other factors in psoriasis that I didn't go into. I tried to speak, to address only one component, that is the vasodilatation, and I mentioned that I think, when I spoke about the use of corticosteroids attacking not just the vasodilatation but also other factors such as the increased rate of growth of the epidermis, the inflammatory component in the dermis, etc. Is that what you're referring to?

PARTICIPANT: Yes. I guess it just is complex and unknown, but the research that I've seen on psoriasis has used warming, not only general, peripheral warming, but also an attempt to warm the specific spots wherever it's located. And the results have been positive with temperature warming which is a little different. You wouldn't expect that to happen with the description you gave of the swollen blood vessels.

MILLER: Is that to change the state of anxiety or is that to affect something very specific physiologically within the psoriatic plaque? Because if it's to change the state of anxiety, then you get completely off the plaque and you run through the whole body again and various other mechanisms may start coming into play.

Because you go back to the brain again and then the brain can shoot
out all the things that it does, including increasing its own corticol output which may then act on the skin or who knows what. That
would be an entirely different situation.

PARTICIPANT: If I understand you, you were suggesting that
vasoconstriction of the psoriatic plaque might be a response taught
with the assistance of biofeedback that perhaps could be helpful for
psoriasis.

MILLER: In that limited fashion, right.

PARTICIPANT: And that's something that is rarely done in
biofeedback circles, vasoconstriction. However there's a good
possibility, except for a temporal artery of migraine headache, that
vasoconstriction has been taught with some benefit. Thank you, Dr.
Miller.

REFERENCES

Adair, J. R., & Theobold, D. E. Raynaud's phenomenon: Treatment of
    a severe case with biofeedback. Journal Indiana State Medical
    Association, 1978, 71 (10), 990-993.
Bird, E. I., & Colborne, G. R. Rehabilitation of an electrical
    burn patient through thermal biofeedback. Biofeedback and
    Self-Regulation, 1980, 5(2), 283-287.
Edelberg, R. Electrical properties of the skin. In C. C. Brown
    (Ed.), Methods in Psychophysiology. Baltimore: Williams &
    Wilkins, 1967.
Haynes, S. N. et al. Biofeedback treatment of atopic dermatitis.
    Controlled case studies of eight cases. Biofeedback and
    Self-Regulation 1979, 4(3), 195-209.
Jacobson, A. M. et al. Raynaud's phenomenon. Treatment with
    hyperotic and operant techniques. Journal of the American
    Medical Association, 1973, 225, 739-740.
Koldys, K. W., & Meyer, R. P. Biofeedback training in the therapy
    of dyshidrosis, Cutis, 1979, 24 (2), 219-221.
Lindsley, D. B., & Sassaman, W. H. Autonomic activity and brain
    potentials associated with "voluntary" control of pilomotors.
    Journal of Neurophysiology, 1938, 1, 342-349.
Miller, R. M., & Coger, R. W. Skin conductance conditioning with
    dyshidrotic eczema patients. British Journal of Dermatology,
    1979, 101 (4), 435-440.
Schleifer, S. J. Bereavement and Lymphocyte function. Paper
    presented to the American Psychiatric Association, San
    Francisco, 1980.
Sappington, J. T. et al. Biofeedback as therapy in Raynaud's
    disease. Review article in Biofeedback and Self-Regulation.
    1979, 4, 155-169.

Tarchanoff, J.   Uber die galvanischen Erscheinungen an der Haut des
    Menschen bei Reizung der Sinnesorgane und die verschiedenen
    Formen dermpsychischer Tätigkeit.   Pflugers Archiv fuer die
    Gesamte Physiologie, 1890, 46, 46-55.
Taub, E., & Stroebel, C. F.   Biofeedback in the treatment of
    vasoconstrictive syndromes.   Biofeedback and Self-Regulation
    1978, 3 (4), 363-373.

PERSONALITY CHARACTERISTICS OF PSYCHOSOMATIC PATIENTS

William H. Rickles

Staff Psychiatrist, Veterans Administration Medical
Center, Sepulveda, California
Associate Research Psychiatrist, Department of
Psychiatry, UCLA Center for the Health Sciences,
Los Angeles, California

Writing a chapter about the personality characteristics of psychosomatic-prone patients poses several difficulties. The main problem arises from the ubiquitous nature of psychosomatic phenomena. To fall ill when stressed is as human as falling in love.

Of course, the degree of stress and severity of illness is a very individual matter, but who among us has never experienced a stress-related disorder of some kind? Thus, to some degree I may be writing about the reader's psychopathology, a subject not dear to the hearts of most physicians and other professionals. Secondly, this chapter is slanted towards physicians. As a group, we are admonished to practice our art in a humanistic way and to treat the "whole patient." Actually, our training does little to foster the realization that a patient's disease is an integral part of the person. In every instance we are encouraged to think of our patients as having their diseases visited upon them. The idea that the disease may be related to (not caused by) the way someone lives his life, and hence that the person is the disease, in part, sounds foreign and metaphysical to medical, scientifically oriented people. Finally, the enormous advances in medical and surgical techniques further obscure the psychosomatic contribution to our patients ills by: (1) strongly impressing the patients, and (2) requiring so much of us to use these pharmacological, surgical, and nuclear tools expertly and safely. Thus we are trained inadvertently to collude with our patients to ignore and often to deprecate psychosomatic relationships.

Accordingly, having acknowledged the difficulties the medical

155

and/or scientific reader may have with this chapter, and having identified myself as a member of both groups, I will proceed in the hope that the foregoing at least will have demonstrated my familiarity with the psyche/soma problem faced by the medical and mental health practitioner.

After briefly reviewing some of the purported difficulties with the older psychoanalytic theories of psychosomatics, I will review a specific and well-studied psychosomatic relationship and follow by describing some of the more general personality characteristics predisposing to stress related psychological breakdown. Concluding with practical therapeutic and referral considerations, I will indicate how well specific and general biofeedback techniques fit the therapeutic requirements of patients with stress-related disorders.

BACKGROUND AND HISTORY

Although useful in individual cases by psychoanalytically trained psychotherapists, the specific theory proposed by Alexander has not found verification in large-scale sociometric studies (Deutch, 1980). Alexander described a unique unconscious conflict associated with each of seven diseases of unknown etiology and postulated these conflicts as pathogenic for the associated disorder (1950). These conditions, often referred to as the "Chicago 7," include peptic ulcer, essential hypertension, bronchial asthma, thyrotoxicosis, rheumatoid arthritis, ulcerative colitis, and neurodermatitis. Since then, psychosomatic research interest has shifted to "psychosocial factors" associated with a much broader range of medical and psychiatric problems. In essence, interest has shifted from the intrapsychic factors in a selected group of conditions to interpersonal influences in virtually all medical conditions. At our present state of knowledge, this shift is appropriate, since the understanding and treatment of unconscious intrapsychic conflict requires extensive training in psychoanalysis and can be applied to relatively few patients. As will be demonstrated, many psychosomatic patients cannot value or understand concepts of disease or therapies aimed at resolving intrapsychic conflict. Further, many serious diseases such as coronary heart disease (CHD) occur in epidemic proportions in the United States (American Heart Association, 1978). Sociopsychological approaches which can yield results translatable into therapies applicable on a large scale are desirable. Clearly, psychoanalysis as a therapeutic modality cannot cope with such large numbers of patients. Still, the findings of the psychoanalytic writers provide concepts which have proven relevant to developing large-scale therapies for stress-related illnesses.

THE TYPE A PERSONALITY

Seventy years ago, in a paper on angina pectoris, Sir William Osler (1910) wrote, "It is not the delicate neurotic person who is prone to angina pectoris, but the robust, the vigorous in mind and body and the keen and ambitious man, the indicator of whose engines is always at 'full speed ahead.'" This vivid and accurate description of the Coronary Heart Disease (CHD) Patient was not dealt with as a clear etiological agent until the 1940s, when Flanders Dunbar (1943), a pioneer in psychosomatic medicine, developed the concept of the "coronary personality." She interviewed several hundred hospital patients and concluded that distinct personality types could be associated with each disease. These findings have been severely challenged, but in the case of the coronary personality described as compulsive, dominating and aggressive, the total evidence supporting or refuting Dunbar is weak and scant (Mattesan & Trancevich, 1980).

Beginning in the 1950s, Freidman and Rosenman (1959) began to operationalize the more abstract concept of a "coronary personality" into specific describable "behavioral patterns" associated with CHD. Their work culminated in the description of a Coronary Prone Behavior Pattern (CPBP) which contributes to the etiology of CHD. In a landmark book (Freidman, 1969), they describe the now renowned Type A behavior pattern as "a characteristic action-emotion complex which is exhibited by those individuals who are engaged in a relatively chronic struggle to obtain an unlimited number of poorly defined things from their environment in the shortest period of time and if necessary, against the opposing effects of other things or persons in the same environment." The pattern has been studied in detail and refined to include (Matteson & Ivanevich, 1980; Suinn, 1977):

1. A perpetual sense of time urgency;

2. Striving to accomplish more and more in less and less time;

3. A driven and competitive attitude;

4. Easily evoked hostility, overt or covert;

5. Chronic impatience;

6. Unease with inactivity or relaxing; and

7. Over value of doing and deprecating of experiencing or being.

Currently, there are two methods of determining the presence of the CPBP: a standard interview (SI) (Rosenman et al., 1964) and the Jenkins Activity Survey (JAS) (Jenkins, Rosenman, & Zyzanski, 1974). Each method has its difficulties, but the ratings agree in 63-91% of the cases (Matteson & Ivanevich, 1980). The range depends largely

on the scores of the JAS. A great deal of research has been
accomplished relating the CPBP to CHD with the following results:

1. In the age group of 39 to 49 years, CPBP in men occasioned
    6.5 times the incidence of CHD than did non-CPBP men
    (Rosenman, 1975).

2. The CPBP is more predictive of CHD than either blood
    pressure, cholesterol, or triglycerides (Rosenman, 1975).

3. CPBP men with CHD were five times more likely to have a
    second infarct than non-CPBP men with CHD (Rosenman, 1975).

4. There is a linear relationship between degrees of CPBP and
    incidences of CHD (Jenkins, Rosenman & Zyzanski, 1974).

5. Significant links between traditional risk factors
    (elevated cholesterol, triglycerides, lipoproteins excre-
    tion or norepinephrine and decreased blood clotting time)
    and CPBP have repeatedly been reported (Mathesan &
    Ivancevich, 1980) but CPBP operates to cause CHD indepen-
    dent of these factors.

Clinical Example

        John is a 53-year-old executive who works for the Air Force as
head of a large aircraft maintainence facility employing over 5000
people. Ten years ago, after a successful career in military avia-
tion, he retired before making general in order to find a civilian
job before he was 50. After a few years as the vice-president of a
parts manufacturing company, he landed the job he had "trained for
all his life," vice-president in charge of maintenance for a major
airline. After an ecstatic year on the job, he was suddenly fired
when all top management positions were filled with new people as a
result of a major reorganization of the company. After unsuccessfully attempting to find a comparable job in private industry, he
took a civil service job which meant that, as a civilian, he
reported to men who previously were junior to him. In addition, he
lost all retirement pay and was in effect working for half pay.
Within one year he developed signs of angina and underwent cardiac
catheterization. Severe coronary artery disease was diagnosed and
four coronary bypass grafts were soon in place.

Arguments and outbursts of hostility often marked his relations with
his wife and four children, who superficially appeared to be an
average, successful middle-class American family. Impatience, com-
petitiveness and inflexible behavior marked his lifestyle. His lack
of psychological awareness was so complete that when asked how he
handled mistakes during a job interview, he replied that he couldn't

answer because he had never made a mistake. He saw these traits as
dedication and caring about things being done right.

Blood pressure and cholesterol have always been normal. He has
never smoked, only had an occasional drink at parties, and spent his
weekends at home working on the yard and other homestead related
projects. None of the usual risk factors could be found in his
medical history other than a strong Type A behavior pattern.

Thus, we may conclude that a lifestyle may have a very profound
influence on the development of serious heart disease. One would be
amazed if this were the only disorder linked to the Type A behavior
pattern, but few studies have been done to examine the relationship
of this pattern to other stress-related medical problems.

ALEXITHYMIA

Simultaneously, the past twenty years have seen another line of
psychosomatic research which has attempted to link the incapacity to
verbalize a range of feeling states to the incidence of serious
psychosomatic disorders. Beginning in the 1960s, Sifneos (1967,
1972) and Nemiah et al. (1978) described the invariant behaviors of
many patients they had been called to see in psychosomatic consultation. They were struck with the frequency with which psychosomatic
patients were unable to describe feelings associated with present
or past events. Further, these patients seemed to appear quite normal in their lifestyles, but had little concept of the nuances of
human interaction. They called this difficulty with the language of
emotion "alexithymia," from the Greek word stem meaning without
words for feelings. Recently, Nemiah (1978) summarized the features
of alexithymia as follows:

1. The vocabulary for emotional expression is severely re-
    stricted to nonspecific expressions such as "nervous" or
    "upset."

2. The bodily sensations often associated with emotion such as
    "a lump in the throat" or "feeling in the chest" or "pit of
    the stomach" do not reach awareness. When sensations are
    present, they usually occur in the region of the patho-
    physiology. For example, an ulcerative colitis patient
    feels a sensation in his "stomach" but indicates the lower
    abdomen with his hand when he is angry.

3. They demonstrate little evidence of experiencing anything
    but extremes of feelings. They often consider themselves
    to be highly emotional because they mistake violent, poorly
    elaborated outbursts of rage or tearfulness as all there is
    to emotion or feelings.

4. Thought content usually is devoid of fantasies related to
    images of feelings or relationships, but is connected with
    the minutiae of external events. For example, when such
    patients are asked to tell about their childhoods, they
    will often say only that "I had a normal, happy childhood."
    Or, when asked to describe her father, one such person
    said, "He is short and dark-haired."

Psychiatric interviews with such patients are either dull and boring
with the interviewer finding that exploring the patient's inner
world is like "pulling hen's teeth," or the patients flood the
interviewer with irrevelent details. Even when nonspecific emotional terms are used, the patient's thinking is clearly stimulus-
bound.

Clinical Example

A 33 year old woman was referred for biofeedback therapy for
her asthma. During the initial interview she made it quite clear
that she had no interest in psychotherapy, but was willing to work
on reducing stress. When the interviewer suggested that she assign
a stress score to each day before she retired, she explained that
this would be pointless, because it would only reflect the number of
stressful events in her day. She was almost incapable of thinking
of stress as an internal experience without relating it to an external stimulus.

5. Patients exhibit a subtle but marked difficulty in talking
    about themselves as experiencing agents. Indefinite pro-
    nouns such as "one", "it," or "you" are used instead of "I"
    when describing an emotional or sensory experience. One
    such patient with a painful and disabling reflex sympathe-
    tic dystrophy of the hand would say, "the hand hurts" or
    "it hurts in the hand" instead of "my hand hurts" or the
    even more personal and subject-active, "I hurt in my hand".
    Sometimes this distancing from self as experiencing agent
    may be extremely subtle and pervasive.

Clinical Example

Bill is a 45-year-old executive who began psychoanalysis for
severe anxiety symptoms which occurred when he moved from vice president to president of a large corporation. During the preceding
year, he had a hemigastrectomy for a perforated duodenal ulcer.
Several psoriatic lesions and chronic, low grade hepatitis had
plagued him for years. Although he reported dreams in profusion,
associated well, and worked on understanding himself, progress was
extremely slow. Only gradually did the manner with which he avoided
self as experiencing agent become apparent. Negative feelings
toward the analyst were either completed before a treatment session

and reported rather than experienced in the session, or he would
wait until an angry response subsided and then refer to the feeling
with remarks such as "there was some anger about that." Attempts to
point out this indirect style were ineffective until his behavior
was characterized as being similar to the women in ancient China who
would point out the location of their complaints on a special doll
carried by the doctor for that purpose. Psychologically, Bill would
create a verbal Chinese doctor's doll during each session which he
would assist me in analyzing and in this way have an analysis
without experiencing it as agent-subject.

    Marty and de M'Uzan (1963) and later de M'Uzan (1974) have
described similar characteristics in their psychosomatic patients.
They note that these patients seldom report dreams. When dreaming
occurs, it usually is without detail and complexity. Under severe
stress, dreams with primitive primary process content may emerge.
They have also described the interpersonal relationships of these
patients as being on the basis of "reduplication." Other people
are seen as duplicates of themselves or as overgeneralized carica-
tures. Thus, interactions are stereotyped and give the appearance
of normality, but are devoid of true empathy.

    McDougall's (1974) benchmark paper expressed these observations
from the point of view of psychosomatic patients. She finds that
psychosomatic patients have a personality deficiency in their ability to symbolize. Without the ability to generate meaning and significance internally, they are driven to external reality to know
what to "think" about an experience. When this reliance on the outside to substitute for internal symbols is extreme, addictive relationships may develop. The result is an extreme vulnerability to
humiliation and disappointment which often precedes psychophysiological breakdown.

Clinical Example

    1. The previously described 33-year-old woman "had always been
        in perfect health" and "never been sick a day" in her life
        prior to the onset of her asthma two years ago. She had
        been working 12 to 16 hours per day starting a business in
        a highly competitive field for approximately 18 months when
        she broke up with her boyfriend. Three weeks of sleep-
        lessness and anorexia followed, which was initially termi-
        nated by a severe case of pneumonia. Recovery from the
        pneumonia was complicated by a persistent asthmatic con-
        dition requiring high doses of steroids and bronchodilators
        and extreme susceptibility to physical or emotional
        stressors.

    2. A 65-year-old woman was severely shaken by the discovery
        that her most adored daughter was homosexual. The next day

she left for a trip to Europe but returned home early after
being hospitalized in London for severe influenza. Headaches and easy fatigability have persisted for two years
and only gradually improved, despite various medical
therapies.

Now we are in a better position to understand why the various
personality assessment instruments have given such inconclusive
results when administered to psychosomatic patients. Because of the
symbolizing deficiency, they largely are denied classical neurotic
defenses. Similarly, the depletion of the inner psychic world
deprives them of psychotic defenses. What may be needed are psychological instruments which are calibrated to measure the capacity to
symbolize and elaborate psychological defenses. Of course, defenses
exist, but as McDougall (1974) notes, the therapist observes facial
movements, gestures, sensory-motor manifestations, or pain at times
when manifestations of neurotic (or psychotic) defenses would be
more likely.

SUMMARY OF ALEXITHYMIA RESEARCH

As interest in this dimension of psychosomatic disorders grows,
a body of research deliniating the difference between alexithymic
and neurotic disorders is developing. However, work is also being
reported which defines the concept on a scientific as well as a
clinical/anecdotal basis. Recently, the Eleventh European
Conference on Psychosomatic Research was devoted to the topic
"Towards a Theory of Psychosomatic Disorders: Alexithymia, Pensee
Operatoire, Psychosomatisches Phenomen." Some of the papers adding
to the validation of the construct will be summarized. Von Rad and
his colleagues (1977) used material gathered from a psychiatric
interview, TAT cards, and a story completion test to compare a group
of neurotic patients to patients with psychosomatic disorders. The
significantly different results include group differences in word
production, use of "I" and "one," therapist interventions, and frequency of affect-laden words. The differences are all consistent
with the psychosomatic patients showing alexithymic behaviors.
Comparable results were achieved in a similar study by Vogt et al.
(1977) and Overbeck (1977).

Alexithymic subjects were less hypnotizable than people who are
better able to express feeling and fantasy (Frankel et al., 1977).
A comparison of irritable bowel syndrome and ulcerative colitis
patients found significantly greater incidence of alexithymics in
the more severely ill, latter group (Fara & Paran, 1977).

Lesser, Ford, and Friedman (1979) used an affect check list
(MAACL) and a sentence completion test to compare psychosomatic and
psychiatric patients. No group differences were found, and they
attributed their finding to the limited verbal skills of their lower

socioeconomic group of subjects. The concept of an alexithymic
syndrome which is independent of other psychopathologic dimensions
is supported by the report by Blanchard, Orena, and Pallmeyer (1981)
which found an alexithymia scale to be statistically independent
from (or orthogonal to) psychometric measures of depression,
hysteria, and anxiety, but highly correlated with incidence of medical disorders.

ETIOLOGY

   Several authors have speculated that a neurophysiological deficit may underlie alexithymic behavior (Nemiah, 1977). McDougall
(1974) presents analytic data suggesting that in addition to organ
specific problems, alexithymic patients were interdicted from
forming transitional object attachments during childhood.

   Transitional objects and their place in childhood development
were first described by Winnicott in 1951 (Winnicott, 1975). Since
then, a considerable literature has developed linking these concepts
to a variety of phenomena (Grolnick & Barkin, 1978). Transitional
objects such as the security blanket or Teddy bear of childhood are
adopted or "discovered" by the child between six and 12 months of
age. The child uses them in place of the mother or thumb as a means
of anxiety reduction and self-soothing. The correlation between
transitional object pathology and a propensity to psychosomatic
breakdown is all the more compelling when we recall that the development of attachments to transitional objects has been found to be
the beginning of the capacity for play and symbolization (Grolnick &
Barkin, 1978). These are the very personality functions which are
problematic in the alexithymic individual. Further, meditation has
been described as "reliably soothing inner experiences with matura-
tional potential" and linked to transitional phenomena (Horton,
1974; Staetz, 1976). McDougall (1974) notes that when describing
their sexual relationships, her psychosomatic patients would either
treat their partners as "feeding mothers upon whom they were des-
perately dependent" or interchangeable sexual partners, but were
highly insistent that someone be there at all times. In either
case, the lover is treated like a "security blanket" who will function like a transitional object. Elsewhere (Rickles, 1976, 1981) I
have suggested that the biofeedback machine may be experienced by
some patients as functioning like a transitional object. A
meditation-like state of mind is required to learn the biofeedback
skill, so in addition to self-regulation of a physiologic system or
symptom, biofeedback assists the patient in acquiring a self-
soothing capability while reestablishing a connection between the
"mind-body team" without threatening the unconscious split between
body feelings and sensations and psychological feelings and
emotions.

   Now it is possible to relate alexithymia to the Type A per-

sonality or CPBP. No direct comparison is presently available, and
no information regarding the dynamics of the CPBP is available.
Some meager information is present in the work of Defourny, Hubin,
and Liminet (1977) which compared the TAT responses of men, classified as Type A and Type B. They found the Type A patients to use
fewer total words in their stories. They had less involvement with
their bodies, treating themselves as batteries which occasionally
needed recharging. Rest was valued only as preparatory for work.
Life was lived assertively in both groups, but the Type A patient
found life dysphoric while the Type B patients found life to be a
pleasure. The stories by Type B patients were like movies which had
a creative, evolving story line, while the Type A patients told static and more stereotypic stories with fewer affective words and more
emotional distance. Further, stories from the Type A patients
revealed difficulties in distinguishing self from others and per-
ceiving the effects of their aggression upon others. Their stories
were more descriptive and perceptive than projective.

In summary, the Type A patients lived their lives according to
stereotypes, ignored their bodily needs; they had a diminished ability to perceive and describe feelings or elaborate fantasy, and they
tended to be more descriptive and operational in their description
of the TAT cards. In all, the Type A patients appear to have many
characteristics of the alexithymia syndrome with considerable
aggressiveness added.

CONCLUSION

The medical patient with a stress-related disorder may fall ill
as the result of homeostatic functioning being overwhelmed at any of
a number of organic and/or psychosocial levels. Recently, George
Engel (1980) related this comprehensive psychosomatic view to general systems theory. The alexithymic syndrome brings together a
number of behavioral and psychodynamic factors which predispose to
psychophysiologic breakdown. Mainly, in the alexithymia syndrome
the patient might be said to be addicted to a stereotyped world of
superficial reality in order to maintain psychophysiologic equilibrium. This "addiction" is invisible to the alexithymic individual
because alternate views threaten this system and are seen as crazy
or foolish. He sees himself as being splendidly self-sufficient and
motivated by circumstantial necessity to do what is either proper or
practical. This cognitive style is obtained at the price of diminished awareness of internal emotional and physical needs. This
diminished awareness is attained by neglecting fantasizing and symbolizing functions. To the psychologically and emotionally receptive observer, the alexithymic appears emotionally superficial,
living like "Humpty Dumpty" in a thin shell of experience between a
symbolically and emotionally empty inner world and a rigid but supportive wall of outer reality. Loss of the supporting wall permits
a shattering "fall" of self-esteem and security. Restoration of the

invulnerable belief system often defies "all the king's horses and all the king's men," including the medical and behavioral science practitioners. Such a "broken" state of illness can drag on for years.

Additionally, the diminished capacity for transforming stressful stimuli into creative thoughts and feelings which may be used to effect self-serving, self-soothing solutions leaves the alexithymic vulnerable to prolonged periods of stress. The body and the personality are subjected to the ill effects of chronic arousal without periodic relief. That is, sometimes the alexithymic syndrome may be responsible for the patient developing the general adaptation syndrome of Selye (1956) and doing so without possibility of detection by most of our psychological sensors!

Treatment Considerations

With development of the concept and characteristics of the alexithymic syndrome, the psychosomatic patient's antipathy towards psychotherapy and psychosomatic concepts become more understandable. The alexithymic is extremely naive concerning intrapsychic experience and identifies all reference to emotional and meaningful intrapsychic experience as implying strangeness, at best, and incompetence, invalidity, and insanity at worst. No wonder the average physician is loathe to suggest psychiatric consultation when such "insults" are inferred by the patient. When psychotherapy is tried, the results are often useless or even negative unless the therapist is sensitive and skilled.

On the more encouraging side, a well defined paradigm to treatment is suggested:

1. The therapist must provide a real world model for the patient because of the alexithymic's extreme dependency on external cues. The modeling will probably be a major mode of change during therapy.

2. Extra effort must be extended to make referral and treatment a narcissistically positive experience.

3. If possible, the therapy should be distributed between several agents. In this way the severe problems in handling ambivalence and psyche/soma integration may be more easily managed (Winnicott, 1966).

4. If possible, the patient's own method of providing self-soothing transitional experiences for himself should be identified and every effort made to stabilize the situation for an optimum availability of these experiences if they are not dangerous or destructive.

5. I have found that educating the patient as to the nature of the problems associated with the alexithymic syndrome greatly facilitates compliance and cooperation. It is extremely important to get some part of the patient to form an alliance with the therapist's concern for the patient's problem of self-regulation and self-care.

6. Depending upon the therapist's orientation, improvement in several personality deficiencies must be approached. Specifically, the patient needs to be helped to improve his capacity to fantasize, empathize, self-observe, recognize feelings/sensations as important signals, and verbalize feelings.

7. Most important, the therapist must go slowly. Outstripping the patient's limited capacity for independent thinking and feeling can cause severe negative therapeutic reactions such as a return of symptoms or breaking off therapy (Winnicott, 1966).

To summarize, I have described the alexithymic syndrome as resulting from a diminished capacity for fantasy and symbolic elaboration. The evolving personality and behavioral constellation includes diminished experiential and verbal emotional life, a superficial interpersonal style with diminished capacity for empathy, vulnerability to narcissistic injury, unacknowledged dependency on others for maintenance of personality equilibrium, and vulnerability to the general adoption syndrome and psychophysiologic breakdown. This model not only is of heuristic value in that it suggests behavioral and developmental antecedents, but predicts important treatment strategies. In closing, I will quote the 18th Century English physician, C. H. Parry, who wrote: "Often, it is much more important to know what sort of patient has a disease than to know what sort of disease a patient has."

DISCUSSION

PARTICIPANT: Sir, have you found any correlation between this alexithymic personality and what we commonly call a sociopathic or psychopathic personality who also frequently has flat affect, no emotional attachment to anyone, no sense of obligation to other people, and is totally self-centered?

RICKLES: I don't know quite how to say this. What we have done is attempt to delineate alexithymia as a dimension. You see, you can define any kind of dimension you want to as long as you define it and are able to quantify it and make it a dimension. Then, it is possible to see all of these kinds of traits in all kinds of patients. The antisocial personality is another dimension

which is not completely orthogonal. None of the other personality
dimensions, such as depression or borderline personality or narcissistic personality, are orthogonal. So these traits will appear
similar to many other things that you have thought about. What
we're trying to do is define this dimension, continuum, because we
think it may have some value in treating and thinking about a propensity to psychophysiological breakdown. So, my answer, in short,
is yes. I think many psychopathic personalities would be alexithymic, but not necessarily all of them. The internal reason for
being, having the same external behavior, may be quite different in
different situations.

PARTICIPANT: Dr. Rickles, has there been any work done with
relation to assessing the different personality traits of children?
If so, can you give me some references? Type A personality?

RICKLES: As far as I know there hasn't been.

PARTICIPANT: Why?

RICKLES: Why? Art is long and life is short. (laughter) Ah,
to back up a little bit, John Lacey did a longitudinal study in
children of motor impulsivity, close to twenty years ago I think,
which might be related if we got into these children a little bit to
some of this and found it to be a stable trait.

PARTICIPANT: Two questions: one psychological and one more
psychoanalytic. The first one, a quicker one: have there been any
correlations between low density lipoprotein/high density lipo-
protein ratios and Type A behavior?

RICKLES: I don't know the answer to that. I haven't gone into
that literature yet that deeply.

FROM AUDIENCE: There were and they were negative.

PARTICIPANT: The other has to do with some continuing work we
are doing trying to correlate certain types of personality traits
with biofeedback success or failure and we're roughly getting two
groups where we have a relatively unexpected success and relatively
expected failure. The unexpected successes are coming in groups of
people who are by and large very seriously personality disturbed,
often borderline people with psychotic histories, and almost always
substance abuse which of course fits into some of the last things
that you were saying. With such people we are finding that marked
deviations from standard biofeedback techniques have been very helpful. We never give tapes. We very rarely give a whole lot of
instruction. We do give some basic relaxation training and then
essentially turn the patient loose to work and control the instrument. We emphasize control a lot; we emphasize relaxation, never.

We find that to emphasize relaxation has been terribly destructive to the treatment process since the patients fear it and, therefore, we never talk about it. But in talking about control and
giving the patient a maximum amount of determination as to what they
do with the instrument, we find an incorporation or control which
then generalizes and extends into outside behavior in a number of
different ways. I think this fits in a lot to what you describe
about trying to activate a transitional object. With the instrument
we consciously attempt to do that, of course, subtly without ever
trying to make it overt. The therapist also becomes the same sort
of phenomenon which we attempt to get the patient to relate to. I
wonder if you might speak at all about this question, these questions, and see if this adds anything to what your own research has
been showing?

RICKLES: I think those are very valuable observations. I
could only reaffirm them, that in many, especially the sicker personalities, more personality disorganized individuals of borderline
types, these are the issues that must be dealt with: control and
permitting maximum autonomy. Because if you intervene too much,
you're going to create a great deal of difficulty. There was some
work many years ago which suggested that low ego strength patients
did much better in biofeedback than high ego strength patients. I
don't know how good that work was, but that was the statement that
was made in one of these meetings.

PARTICIPANT: That is precisely our finding, that the low ego
strength patients were doing much better. The other group, which we
were spectacularly unsuccessful with, were the people with very high
ego strength which largely fell into the alexithymic, obsessive-
compulsive type categories that you were describing.

RICKLES: However, we think that obsessive-compulsive traits
are different from alexithymia. They have fantasies, that's a
neurotic defense behind them. Alexithymia doesn't.

PARTICIPANT: As you were describing the alexithymic personality, I was visualizing that type of patient that I see in my
office as a primary care physician and I never bothered to think of
it in that way before. But sort of formulating the kind of strategy
that I would employ to deal with that sort of patient whom I see as
coming in with a set of symptoms and a set of restrictions and pro-
scriptions in hand about what he or she will and will not allow to
be done about this, and also coming in as if he were taking himself
to the doctor. This is my brother, me. The strategy that I think
I use, in fact, and I'd like you to comment on it--the question
is, would you comment on it in terms of the personality type, in
terms of its validity--is, I say to a patient like that, "This guy
over here needs these things done to him and I know it takes
courage--which it does for that kind of person--courage and

determination to do that to this guy, and I respect the hell out of you for making the attempt that I know you are about to make." But not "You need this stuff done because you've got the following problems." Rather, he has the following problems and I sort of trade on that and suggest that the person is quite brave for attempting to deal with his substance abuse and his pain and his thises and thats. I just wonder if you might comment on the kind of approach of the primary care pre-psychiatric referral physicians in dealing with these kinds of patients?

RICKLES: You would have done well in play therapy (laughter). Exactly. You've got the point and you've discovered the point I am making in your own framework - the part of the transitional object. What's so important is that mother and father go along with the illusion. The development of the capacity to make illusion, to form illusions for oneself, which one can then feel safe within, is extremely important. The patients need, if the child says, "Teddy was bad today. I'm going to spank him." The parents must not say, "That's just a Teddy bear. How can it be bad or good? It's just a little stuffed animal." That's not the way to do it. The way to do it is say "Yeah, what did he do? Why was he so bad? Well, you better give him a spanking." Or you might suggest some better methods of handling it, for the child may take them in or he may not. See, all these things now go into the mind and they come out in adult verbal behavior. But the concept of the transitional experience and the transitional object, I find, is very, very useful in thinking about these funny ways that people talk about themselves. So talking about this other person that he's brought in, his Teddy bear self, that he can talk about and then you just collude with him in the illusion and say "Right, we're going to do something for him." I think it's very right. Thanks.

PARTICIPANT: To back space to the Type A personality material again, I am aware that several years ago Friedman and Rosenman were undertaking a rather ambitious study in terms of trying to alter Type A behavior and I haven't run across anything in the literature about that. Do you happen to know any outcomes from that? I know they were dividing a large number of Type A personalities into reasonably typical groups and then trying to work with a number of different behavior modification techniques in an effort to see if they could indeed effect both personality changes and the longterm morbidity and mortality rates.

RICKLES: No, I am not familiar with the outcome of that work.

PARTICIPANT: Dr. Rickles, can you describe briefly the comparison between hypomanic personality or that trait and Type A behavior?

RICKLES: I think, again, this is another dimension. The hypo-

manic personality is based on manic defenses. Again you see, it
depends on what the internal experience is. What the basis of the
behavior is makes a lot of difference, I think, in what some of the
results will be. A hypomanic personality is based on manic defenses
and we didn't have a chance to go into what manic defenses are.
Basically, manic defenses are a whole series of defenses aimed at
eradicating internal meaningful psychological experience. Roughly
speaking. So the hypomanic personality that is based on manic
defense rather than on need to get a certain deadline taken care of
and then going back to basic rest and self-care situation is one
thing. But if this is a personality defense structure, I think it
is very similar to and very closely related to the Type A personality, and may very well have many alexithymic characteristics.
Remember, this is a syndrome that we're beginning to pull together a
concept of and all of the proper defining features. I'm not sure
that we have them all yet, at all, but we are beginning to do some
research on that.

PARTICIPANT: Dr. Rickles, with this new definition, would you
have anything to say to grade school teachers about prevention of
alexithymia? Should we work on fantasy more?

RICKLES: I have a problem with that question. It's a purely
personal bias and that is that you have so little input to the grade
school student. I have done a lot of thinking about this, but I
think it's mainly a bias. You have so little input to the grade
school student compared to the home environment that I don't think
that what you do does much good.

PARTICIPANT: I have more of a plea than a question, I think,
but I hope you'll comment on my plea and as a partially . . .

RICKLES: You're not guilty.

PARTICIPANT: O.K., guilty of being a partially modified Type
A, alexithymic family physician working in Silicon Valley, where I
think 50% of our practice are the kind of people you are describing.
I am thinking two things. One, that a great deal of creativity is
needed in private practice to deal with the patients that we see,
and understanding that a very strong development of the scientific
base of what we are doing is absolutely necessary to work from. The
creativity aspect of what we are doing is what we don't hear a lot
about in these meetings. What you're saying is so extremely important, I think, that I make a plea that you, either you or people who
make up the program, would spend more time on the very thing that
you are doing. Because I think in our practice, where I use biofeedback on some of my own patients and referred patients from other
physicians, we've come to think of the biofeedback therapist instrument, machine, whatever, as a transitional object. That we, in a
sense, are people who have wavy arms we use hypnosis with, because

these people very easily go into trances doing biofeedback and that sort of thing. But I would like to hear a lot more, is all I'm saying, of the kind of thing you are talking about.

RICKLES: Well, that's lecture number two about the psycho-dynamics of biofeedback in which we relate the biofeedback machines to the transitional object.

REFERENCES

Alexander, F. Psychosomatic medicine, its principles and applications. New York: W.W. Norton, 1950.

American Heart Association. Heart facts reference sheet. Dallas: American Heart Association Communications Divisions, 1978.

Blanchard, E. B., Arena, J. G., & Pallmeyer, T. P. The psychometric properties of a scale to measure alexithymia. Psychotherapy and Psychosomatics (in press).

Defourney, M., Hubin, P., & Luminet, D. Alexithymia, "pensee operatoire" and predisposition to coronopathy pattern "A" of Friedman and Rosenman. Psychotherapy and Psychosomatics, 1977, 27, 106-114.

Deutsch, L., Psychosomatic medicine from a psychoanalytic viewpoint. Journal of the American Psychoanalytic Association, 1980, 28, 653-702.

de M'Uzan, M. Psychodynamic mechanisms in psychosomatic symptom formation. Psychotherapy and Psychosomatics, 1974, 23, 103-110.

Dunbar, F. Psychosomatic diagnosis. New York: Hoeber Press, 1943.

Engel, G. L. The clinical application of the biopsychosocial model. American Journal of Psychiatry, 1980, 137, 535-544.

Fava, G. A., & Pavan, L. Large bowel disorders. II. Psycho-pathology and alexithymia. Psychotherapy and Psychosomatics, 1976-1977, 77, 100-105.

Frankel, F. et al. The relationship between hypnotizability and alexithymia. Psychotherapy and Psychosomatics, 1977, 28, 172-178.

Friedman, M. & Rosenman, R. H. Association of specific behavior pattern with blood and cardiovascular findings. Journal of the American Medical Association, 1959, 169, 1286.

Friedman, M. Pathogenesis of coronary artery disease. New York: McGraw Hill, 1969.

Grolnick, S. A., Barkin, L., Muensterberger, W. Between reality and fantasy: Transitional objects and phenomena. In S.A. Grolnick, L. Barkin, & W. Muensterberger (Eds.), Between fantasy and reality: The transitional object. New York: Jason Aronson, 1978.

Horton, P. C. The mystical experiences: Substances of an illusion, Journal of the American Psychoanalytic Association, 1974, 22(2), 364-380.

Jenkins, C. D., Rosenman, R. H., & Zyzanski, S. J. Prediction of
    clinical coronary heart disease by a test for the coronary-
    prone behavior pattern. New England Journal of Medicine, 1974,
    290, 1271-1275.

Lesser, I. M., Ford, C. V., & Friedman, C. T. H. Alexithymia in
    somatizing patients. General Hospital Psychiatry, 1979,
    256-261.

Marty, P., & de M'Uzan, M. La pensee operatoire, Revue Francaise
    de Psychoanalyse, 1963, 27:suppl, 1345-1356.

Matteson, M. T., & Ivancevich, J. M. The coronary-prone behavior
    pattern: A review and appraisal. Social Science and Medicine,
    1980, 14A, 337-351.

McDougall, J. The psychosoma and psychoanalytic process.
    International Review of Psycho-Analysis, 1974, 1, 437-459.

Nemiah, J. C., Freyberger, H., & Sifneos, P. E. Alexithymia: A
    view of the psychosomatic process. In O. Hill (Ed.), Modern
    trends in psychosomatic process. London/Boston: Butterworth,
    1976.

Nemiah, J. Alexithymia and psychosomatic illness. Journal of
    Continuing Education in Psychiatry, 1978, 25-37.

Osler, W. Angina pectoris. Lancet, 1980, 2, 839.

Overbeck, G. How to operationalize alexithymic phenomena-some
    findings from speech analysis and the Giesser test (GT).
    Psychotherapy and Psychosomatics, 1977, 28, 106-117.

Rickles, W. H. Biofeedback, therapy, and transitional phenomena
    of psycho-somatic/narcissistic disorders. Psychiatric Annals,
    1981, 11(3), 23-41.

Rickles, W. H. Some theoretical aspects of the psychodynamics of
    successful biofeedback therapy. Journal of Biofeedback and
    Self-Regulation, 1976, 1, 348.

Roseman, R. H., Brand, R. J., Jenkins, C. D., Friedman, M., Straus,
    R., & Wurm, M. Coronary heart disease in the Western collo-
    borative group study: Final follow-up experience of 8-1/2
    years. Journal of the American Medical Association, 1975, 233,
    872.

Rosenman, R. H., Friedman, M., Straus, R., Wurm, M., Kostitchek,
    R., Hahn, W., & Werthessen, N. T. A predictive study of coro-
    nary heart disease. Journal of the American Medical
    Association, 1964, 189, 103.

Sifneos, P. Clinical observations in some patients suffering from
    a variety of psychosomatic diseases. Proceedings of the 7th
    European Conference of Psychosomatic Research, 1967, 73, 339.

Sifneos, P. E. The prevalence of "alexithymic" characteristics in
    psychosomatic patients. In H. Freyberger (Ed.), Topics of
    Psychosomatic Research, Basle, Karger, 1972.

Straetz, M. R. Transitional phenomena in the treatment of ado-
    lescents. Contemporary Psychoanalysis, 1976, 12, 507-513.

Suinn, R. M. Type A behavior pattern. In R. B. Williams & W. D.
    Gentry (Eds.), Behavioral approaches to medical treatment.
    Cambridge: Ballinger Publishing Co., 1977.

Vogt, R. et al. Differences in phantasy life of psychosomatic and
     psychoneurotic patients. Psychotherapy and Psychosomatics,
     1977, 28, 98-105.
Von Rad, M., Lalucat, L., & Lolas, F. Differences of verbal behav-
     ior in psychosomatic patients. Psychotherapy and Psycho-
     somatics, 1977, 28, 83-95.
Winnicott, D. W. Transitional objects and transitional phenomena.
     In D. W. Winnicott, Through paediatrics to psycho-analysis:
     The collected papers of D. W. Winnicott. New York: Basic
     Books, 1975.

BIOFEEDBACK AND MEDICINE

David S. Gans

Medical Director
Sandweiss Biofeedback Institute
Beverly Hills, California

INTRODUCTION

Biofeedback is a relatively new therapeutic modality that is showing increasing promise in the treatment of a wide variety of illnesses and symptom complexes. Initially viewed as a way of achieving stress reduction and alleviating "psychosomatic" symptoms, biofeedback is proving useful in an ever-expanding group of specific medical circumstances. The efficacy of biofeedback in treating these illnesses and symptom complexes raises many questions, both as to their pathophysiology and as to what might be unique to the process of biofeedback.

This chapter will address itself to the following topics:

1. A description of biofeedback and a few general comments;

2. Specific uses for biofeedback in medicine;

3. A general discussion of biofeedback as a therapeutic modality; and

4. Some considerations important to the clinical practice of biofeedback.

SECTION I - A DESCRIPTION OF BIOFEEDBACK

It would be helpful to advance some sort of description of biofeedback that is salient to clinical medicine. Biofeedback has been described in a variety of ways. Descriptions, some perjora-

175

tive, such as "mumbo jumbo," or "placebo," and some more accurate,
such as "relaxation training with machines," "education,"
"conditioning," "teaching control of the autonomic nervous system,"
"Western meditation," are interesting, but not clinically useful.
Clinical medicine requires a description of biofeedback that allows
evaluation, in various clinical circumstances, as to both its utility and toxicity.

Biofeedback could be described as a therapeutic modality, or
family of modalities, which attempts to produce in a patient the
ability to control certain physiologic processsess. The means to do
this involve monitoring these processes in the patient and
displaying signals generated from such monitoring to the therapist
and to the patient. The therapist uses a variety of techniques to
facilitate the acquisition of this control. To date, biofeedback
does not employ surgical or pharmacological adjuncts to achieve its
end. A biofeedback therapist is someone trained in the use of this
therapeutic tool in some or all of its applications.

One of the greatest strengths of medicine as it is currently
practiced is its rigid empiricism. Medicine will rightly demand
this of biofeedback. Biofeedback may be evaluated on three levels
as to its efficacy. First, can biofeedback provide a patient with
control over any displayed physiological parameters? Second, can
biofeedback provide a patient with the ability to control a physiological parameter that is not being displayed? Third, and most
important, does this ability to control these parameters achieve a
resolution of the symptom complex or problem for which the patient
sought biofeedback, and is this resolution linked to the control of
the physiological process? This type of evaluation would allow a
comparison of one type of biofeedback to another in any given
problem, and also allows biofeedback to be compared to other forms
of therapy for any given problem. Such evaluations are critical if
biofeedback is to find its appropriate medical uses.

SECTION II - CURRENT MEDICAL USES IN BIOFEEDBACK

Biofeedback is already established as a primary treatment in
several conditions and a promising and/or useful adjunctive treatment in many others. Although more evaluation is necessary, there
are controlled studies in support of these contentions. Larger,
more complete studies will be forthcoming pending time, money, and
medical interest.

For the purposes of this chapter, "primary modality" means an
appropriate first choice of treatment. "Adjunctive therapy" means
an established useful treatment modality, which cannot yet, or may
never, be generally regarded as a primary therapy. These are determinations that require evaluating the efficacy and the safety of

competitive therapies vis-a-vis biofeedback. In general, biofeedback is much safer than the pharmacological and/or surgical
alternatives.

Headache

Biofeedback is a primary treatment modality in moderate or
severe migraine syndromes. Biofeedback has a well-documented cure
rate of 75% with no demonstrable adverse effects (Sandweiss et al.,
1982; Werbach, 1978; Sargent et al., 1973). Decisions about treatment certainly involve accomplishing the therapeutic goal in the
safest, least costly manner possible. If a healthy young individual
has two migraines a year that respond rapidly to a small dose of
ergotamine, which he or she can take without a problem, that would
seem to be the preferred treatment. An individual, on the other
hand, who requires Propanalol, ergots, and analgesics on an ongoing
basis would be given a trial biofeedback. Werbach and Sandweiss
(1978) have demonstrated that both temperature training and relaxation training are about equally effective, although temperature
training is generally employed.

Biofeedback enjoys excellent success with tension headaches
(Sargent, Green, & Walters, 1973; Matulich, Ruch, & Perlis, 1978).
Whether these are in fact a distinct pathological entity need not
concern us here. There is yet no specific physiologic process identified in muscle contraction headaches. Rather, they are treated
nonspecifically with analgesics, tranquilizers, muscle relaxants and
prostoglandin inhibitors. The toxicity of these agents and their
lack of specificity make them a rather poor treatment. Biofeedback
is at present the safest and most efficacious treatment available
for these headaches. Frontalis and trapezius EMG are generally
employed. The cure rate in most controlled studies involving
"muscle contraction" headaches is 75 to 80%.

Raynaud's Disease

The pharmacological and surgical treatent for Raynaud's disease
has significant risks. In both anecdotal reports and group studies,
it has been shown that biofeedback can ameliorate Raynaud's phenomena in 70% of patients (Sedlacek, 1979; Gerber, 1979), with good
maintenance, up to one year in those patients who had follow-up.
The studies have not always distinguished between primary and secondary Raynaud's, a difference which intuitively seems important,
and the follow-up has been variable. Nevertheless, considering our
treatment alternatives, biofeedback, until further notice, has an
excellent claim as a treatment which currently should be considered
first. Temperature feedback is used in this instance.

Fecal Incontinence
<u>Fecal Incontinence</u>

    In those patients with fecal incontinence who have an intact
efferent limb to their external anal sphincter, and who have reasonably intact mentation, biofeedback training using balloon catheters
has been very successsful. A rectal balloon is inflated, producing
rectal distention. Internal sphincter relaxation then occurs. The
patients were trained using an external sphincter balloon to
contract their external anal sphincters in response to lessening
degrees of rectal stimulation. The "n" for this procedure is now
quite large (Engel, Nikoomanesh, & Shuster, 1974; Cerulli,
Nikoomanesh, & Shuster, 1976). There are well-constructed studies
in which these procedures have been employed in a wide variety of
conditions producing fecal incontinence. The patients were followed
up to 22 months, after a brief training period with 72% good
response ("n" equals 36). Fifty-six per cent of the good responders
had no incontinence. Twenty-eight percent had less than one episode
monthly, and 16% had a 90% decrease in the number of episodes.
Considering the surgical alternatives, if this type of biofeedback
training is available, it would seem mandatory that the rectally
incontinent patient be given a trial of biofeedback first.

    Biofeedback is proving an important adjunctive therapy in a
wide variety of conditions:

    (1) Hypertension;

    (2) Bruxism;

    (3) Dysmenorrhea/obstetrics;

    (4) Claudication;

    (5) Stuttering;

    (6) Seizure disorders;

    (7) Functional gastrointestinal disorders;

    (8) Chronic anxiety;

    (9) Stroke rehabilitation;

    (10) Spasmodic torticollis; and

    (11) Stress reduction.

Biofeedback has also shown promise in the treatment of:

    (1) Cardiovascular disorders;

(2) Asthma;

(3) Substance abuse;

(4) Diabetes; and

(5) Hyperactivity and learning disabilities.

Many of these uses are "adjunctive" because there is not yet
a sufficiently large body of work to unequivocally advocate biofeedback as the appropriate clinical response to these problems. The
evidence to date, however, clearly points in this direction in many
of these areas. Many of the studies, although not conclusive, are
quite dramatic and exciting.

Biofeedback is showing increasing documented efficacy in the
treatment of hypertension. Originally viewed three or four years
ago as an "interesting" but basically ineffective adjunctive treatment in a labile Type A hypertension, biofeedback is now producing
dramatic sustained blood pressure drops in moderate and severe
hypertensives (Fahrion, 1979). Although there is, as yet, a lack of
conclusive replicability in biofeedback treatment of hypertension
(Fahrion, 1979; Blanchard & Fahrion, 1978), biofeedback has, at
least in some instances, produced dramatic blood pressure drops.
Significant medication reductions including medication free normo-
tension with major medication usage pretreatment have also been
reported (Fahrion, 1979; Sedlacek, 1976). There have also been
demonstrated drops in Cortisol and VMA levels in biofeedback treated
hypertensives (McCrady, Tan, Crane, & Fine, 1979).

Bruxism is a prominent component of the temporomandibular
joint syndrome. While biofeedback cannot resolve anatomical joint
and dental problems, it is of great value in the treatment of
bruxism (Carlsson, Gale, & Ohman, 1975; Budzinski & Stoyva, 1973).

In dysmenorrhea and obstetrics, biofeedback has already shown
some promise. Dysmenorrhea has been treated by Tubbs and Carnahan
with EMG frontalis muscle training and hand temperature training
(Tubbs & Carnahan, 1976). They reported a 40 to 50% good response.
Sedlacek reports up to 83% good response adding direct vaginal temperature training (Sedlacek & Heczey, 1977). A small vaginal probe
is used after initial familiarization with biofeedback techniques
and the patient is taught to raise vaginal temperature. This has
the above-noted effect in terms of aborting dysmenorrheal cramping.
Self-administered biofeedback at home (small portable EMG and GSR
meters were used) significantly shortened first stage labor time and
reduced medication requirements in both primiparas and multiparas
(Gregg, 1975).

Neuromuscular Disorders

Biofeedback has also been shown to be of great help in certain
neuromuscular dysfunctions. This use of biofeedback is highly specialized and cannot be adequately administered in the usual clinical
setting. Biofeedback has been used in the control of stuttering and
has been highly effective. Biofeedback has also been used in
seizure disorders. This involves a special type of feedback and is
a highly specialized use of this therapeutic modality. Its use has
allowed patients with convulsive disorders to reduce, or, in some
cases, discontinue their medication. This promises to be of great
help in those cases when the patient is experiencing unreasonable
levels of toxicity from "polypharmacy" which is required to control
his or her seizures (Shabsin, Bahler, & Lubar, 1978; Lubar et al.,
1979). Biofeedback has also been used in a highly specialized way
in peripheral nerve disorders following trauma, and paresis secondary to central nervous system damage, for example, following
cardiovascular accident or stroke. EMG is used in a highly specialized way in these cases and has been proven to be quite
effective. Such uses have also been transposed to patients with
cerebral palsy and have been shown to exceed physiotherapy in their
rehabilitative potential (Mandel & Sharp, 1979; Rubow & Netsell,
1979; Koheil, Mandel, & Iles, 1979). While biofeedback promises to
be a very useful and exciting new therapeutic modality in these
areas, it is also clearly a specialized modality which will be
employed by those people involved in rehabilitating the neuromuscu-
larly disabled patient, and will not be a generally available
technique, at least for the forseeable future.

Biofeedback has also been shown to be of value in other types
of chronic muscular disorders such as a spasmodic torticollis
blepharospasm and strabismus (Jankel, 1978; Jensen & Stoffer, 1978).

Claudication

Treadmill walking time in patients with peripheral vascular
disease (N = 11) was markedly improved by (Greenspan et al., 1980).
Pretreatment distances of less than two-tenths of a mile were
increased to one and an eighth miles at six weeks in seven out of
eleven patients. These distances were sustained over six months of
follow-up. The other four patients at least doubled their walking
distance. This was accomplished with a slight reduction in
brachiosystolic blood pressure. In addition, the patient's
tolerance to walking was increased at about the same ankle blood
pressure pre- and postbiofeedback, indicating that this was not
merely due to increased pain tolerance. EMG followed by temperature
training was used (Greenspan & Lawrence, 1980).

Stress Reduction

Biofeedback has been used in a variety of situations for stress and anxiety reduction. These situations have been associated with occupation-related debilitating physical illness, psychological problems, and those cases where people identify themselves only as wishing "to be able to relax more." In all these cases, structured stress and anxiety reduction has proven to be very effectively achieved with biofeedback, with essentially no negative side effects. It is probably least effective in those cases with associated chronic debilitating illness, where it appears that the most important variable for reducing anxiety and depression is that of improving the physical disability. Many high-stress occupations, businesses and institutions now employ biofeedback for this purpose (Hiebert & Fitzsimmons, 1979).

Gastrointestinal Disease

Biofeedback is beginning to be used in a variety of gastrointestinal disorders. These studies are somewhat preliminary, but are quite promising in some cases. In one series of studies, small groups of subjects have been taught to vary their rate of gastric acid secretion. Duodenal ulcer patients using general relaxation training have had improvement in both subjective and uncontrolled objective parameters in terms of both symptomatic relief and ulcer healing (Aleo & Nicassio, 1978; Gorman, 1976). Playing the patient's irritable bowel sounds back to him or her produced improvement in irritable bowel syndrome (Furman, 1973). Other investigators have had similar results with intraluminal balloons and/or general relaxation training (Bueno-Miranda, Cerulli, & Shuster, 1976). These studies are small, not always well-controlled, and not always replicated. They do, however, show promise.

Cardiovascular Disease

Biofeedback has also shown initial utility in the treatment of cardiovascular disease. Greenspan has worked with Type A cardiac patients improving their rehabilitation. Reis, Weiss and others have had some success with a limited number of patients with cardiac arrhythmias, supraventricular as well as premature ventricular contractions (Greenspan & Lawrence, 1980). In an especially exciting communique, C. H. Hartman (1979) taught left hand warming to three chronic angina patients who then reported an ability to abort or control anginal episodes with this technique. The response is quite dramatic, one patient going from 7 nitrobid and 20 or so nitroglycerine a day to no nitrates of any kind (Hartman, 1979).

Substance Abuse

     Biofeedback has been used in substance abuse with mixed
results. It is generally felt by the investigators, however, that
biofeedback may add something to the treatment of alcoholics and
other substance abusers (Reinking, 1978; Marlatt, Rose, Pagano, &
Marques, 1978).

Pulmonary Disease

     Biofeedback has been used in controlled studies to alleviate
bronchospasm in bronchitis and chronic obstructive lung disease.

Diabetes

     The study by Shavoy which showed that biofeedback can cause
blunting of catecholamine responses has interesting implications for
insulin dependent diabetics (Shavoy, Williams, & Johnson, 1979).
There have been anecdotal reports suggesting that diabetic patients
with high degrees of anxiety and stress who undertake biofeedback
begin to require insulin reductions to avoid hypoglycemic shock.

Learning Disabilities

     Investigators and workers in the area of behavioral and
learning disablities have used biofeedback with hyperkinesis and
various types of learning disablilities. The results in these cases
have been equivocal with both EMG and EEG biofeedback being used
(Baldwin, Benjamins, Meyers, & Grant, 1978; Cunningham & Murphy,
1978; Jeffrey, 1978; Kay, Shiverly, & Kilkenny, 1978; Patmon &
Murphy, 1978). In some cases with learning disabled children, some
learning ability in some areas was increased; in other areas it was
not. In hyperkinetic children, there were variable results. The
hyperkinetic children showed a variable degree of improvement in
both hyperkinetic behavior and learning ability in the classroom.
These studies were by no means conclusive but point out an area
where further investigation is required. Biofeedback has also been
used in very young preschool and first grade children who are not
defined as disabled in any way. Interesting results (as compared to
control groups), both in terms of ability to relax and to lengthen
attention span, were achieved, although there was some variability
in results (Hughes & Collins, 1978; Engelhardt, 1978). In spite of
the variability, the promise shown by this program has been such
that in South Dakota several other public schools have adopted it.
While this may not seem an appropriate role in medicine, it is an
interesting application.

SECTION III - BIOFEEDBACK AS A THERAPEUTIC MODALITY,   GENERAL
DISCUSSION

There is an old adage in medicine, "any therapy powerful enough
to benefit is powerful enough to cause harm." Biofeedback is,
however, one of those therapies that, when employed properly, has a
very low potential for damage. This is reflected in the scant
number of contraindications to biofeedback. It is to be expected
that with more sophisticated biofeedback techniques and increased
use of biofeedback in general, more problems will arise. To date,
there are no absolute contraindications to biofeedback, and few
relative contraindications.

Biofeedback should not be used for an unevaluated symptom
complex. One of the effects of biofeedback is that it almost always
produces an enhanced feeling of general well-being (APA Task Force,
1980). This can produce a degree of symptom amelioration no matter
what the cause. This can allow a process which requires a different
type of therapy to go untreated. For example, headache, unevaluated, is not appropriate for biofeedback. The patient may feel
better with biofeedback, and thus wait several weeks before treating
his or her meningioma. Biofeedback is a medical therapy and
requires, for its safe and effective application, a pretreatment
medical evaluation. There are one or two psychiatric conditions
which present relative contraindications to biofeedback. The schizophrenic and severe depressive disorders have both been characterized as disorders in which the patient has to increase his
defences against the grave disruption of his cognitive or affective
processes. In these cases, biofeedback has been of little value
(Marcus & Legin, 1977). Indeed, induced relaxation may prove
harmful. Moderate or situational depression is not a contraindication to biofeedback.

Cognitive impairment of a sufficient degree to interfere with
an understanding of the biofeedback process can preclude successful
treatment. Minor degrees of impairment, when combined with
rigidity, will have the same effect. For this and perhaps other
reasons, elderly patients often do not do well with biofeedback.
There have been interesting results, however, when viewing biofeedback as operant conditioning with retarded children. By using
rewards for success in manipulating desired physiological
parameters, otherwise "unreachable" children have been effectively
treated with biofeedback (Finley, 1979).

Certainly, if a patient views biofeedback with apprehension and
at the same time has an illness that can be adversely affected by
acute anxiety (e.g., acute myocardial infarction), biofeedback
should be deferred. As biofeedback therapy becomes more widespread
and sophisticated, other contraindications are bound to arise. For
example, one would not like to "train" a patient with premature

ventricular contractions and a normal pulse rate to ablate those premature ventricular contractions by learning to maintain a persistent
sinus tachycarrhythmia. As yet, however, there are relatively few
contraindications to biofeedback. In general, when any given illness or symptom complex is amenable to biofeedback therapy, it offers
a safer therapy than the pharmacological or surgical alternatives.

An important controversy and/or confusion surrounding biofeedback centers on whether it is a psychotherapeutic or a medical
treatment modality, both in terms of its administration and in terms
of what it is used to treat. This controversy has important practical implications and should be addressed.

Those "on the side" of psychotherapy maintain that most, if not
all, diseases treated by biofeedback are "psychosomatic" or (often
this appears interchangeable) "stress related" or "psychophysiologic." Therefore, it is argued, biofeedback is the province of the
skilled psychotherapist and should be practiced under his or her
license.

In opposition to this, the author would argue that "psychosomatic" or "psychophysiologic" disease is a term that lacks a precise or useful definition. The usual notion appears to be that
intrapsychic conflicts or "dysfunctional" intrapsychic mechanisms
used in dealing with external experiences produce physical disease.
Certainly, stress as defined by Selye and others can reduce host
resistance and adversely influence the course of an illness.
Certainly, human beings exhibit a multitude of behavioral patterns
that produce disease, injury, or death (substance abuse, violence,
suicide, refusal to seek aid for physical disability, etc.) But
neither stress nor these functional behaviors, both of which are
objectively verifiable, qualify as psychosomatic disease. While the
notion of a psychosomatic disease may be enticing, it enjoys no
objective proof or even any operationally useful definition.
Further, there is no good evidence that psychotherapy is effective
in resolving any of these illnesses referred to as psychosomatic
(Rickles, 1979). Most of the conditions discussed in this chapter
as treatable with biofeedback are not commonly held to be psychosomatic. Psychotherapeutic uses of biofeedback are quite real.
They do not, however, constitute a major area of its applicability.
Biofeedback has been used for stress reduction in a wide variety of
circumstances with excellent results. Any primary care physician
should, however, in the vast majority of such cases, be able to
identify the problem and initiate an appropriate referral. Many of
these patients are, in fact, inappropriate and unwilling candidates
for psychotherapy. While stress reduction could certainly be
labeled a psychotherapeutic use of biofeedback, it should not be
employed only by psychotherapists. Biofeedback is an excellent
substitute for most minor tranquilizer prescriptions that last more
than a month or so. Certainly, most of these prescriptions are not

initiated by psychotherapists.

Biofeedback has been shown to be of benefit in reducing anxiety
in inpatient psychiatric populations (Hiebert & Fitzsimmons, 1979).
Those populations presumably did not have major psychoses, but were
defined as medically and legally able to give consent for biofeedback therapy. Biofeedback has also been shown to be of some use as
an adjunct to family therapy. This use, however, was not controlled
enough to state with certainty that this is a unique contribution
that biofeedback makes in family therapy. Biofeedback and substance
abuse could be viewed as a quasi-psychotherapeutic use, but not
strictly so. Further, as mentioned before, it is not clear as to
what degree this is a beneficial adjunctive use.

The use of biofeedback in a wide variety of symptom complexes
and disease states, cutting across many medical subspecialities, is,
on the other hand, growing rapidly and producing empirically verifiable results. This can only support the author's contention that
biofeedback is showing its greatest potential as a medical therapy,
as opposed to a psychotherapy. The APA has supported this contention, at least to the extent that it has found biofeedback to be of
very little benefit as a psychotherapeutic tool (APA Task Force,
1980).

As a therapeutic modality, biofeedback has one other
interesting and often important difference from conventional pharma-
cologic and surgical alternatives. These later therapies basically
make the practitioner (actively) responsible for healing the
(passive) patient. Some patients, for reasons of secondary gain,
"refuse" to get well. The practitioner is then at fault for
"failing to cure the patient." Biofeedback is, in a way, an educational process. The patient is taught to control certain physiological parameters. Sometimes, as with any therapy, successful
control does not always alleviate the problem. Refusal to work for
achieving this control, however, usually spells certain failure and
is also usually the patient's doing. This can force the patient to
accept the responsibility for participating in his or her cure. If
nothing else, it can be of great comfort to the beleaguered
practitioner.

SECTION IV - THE CLINICAL PRACTICE OF BIOFEEDBACK

The first questions that should be answered in this section
are, "Who does biofeedback?" and "Who should do biofeedback?"
Currently, biofeedback is practiced by three groups of individuals.

The first group consists of individuals with no demonstrable
training who have simply purchased the requisite instruments and set
up shop. These operations are, thankfully, infrequent, as insurance

companies will not compensate such individuals. In general, they
are dangerous, as they offer biofeedback for any symptom, evaluated
or not, and will treat anyone willing to pay. The lack of adequate
licensure provisions paves the way for the existence of such
quackery. Most health care professionals have had their unprin-
cipled advertisements inflicted upon them in several of the "now
generation" publications.

The second group consists of individuals who have been certified as competent providers of biofeedback therapy. Practitioners
in this group may or may not be otherwise licensed health care professionals (for example, physicians, clinical psychologists,
registered physiotherapists, etc.). If licensed, they may practice
biofeedback under that license and receive insurance payments.
Those therapists who are certified but not licensed must, to be eli-
gible for insurance compensation, practice under someone else's
license. Certification is currently performed, generally in good
faith, by the Biofeedback Certification Institute of America or
state organizations. Such certification usually requires completion
of both a practical and didactic training period and completion of
both a practical and written exam. While these societies have
ethics committees and peer review provisions, certification is still
a far cry from state licensure.

A third group of practitioners are those individuals who are
not certified, but are licensed health care professionals in other
areas. They practice biofeedback under their license. Their
training and background is variable.

The following paragraphs are my speculations and proposals concerning biofeedback licensure.

Biofeedback currently costs about $40.00 to $70.00 per hour.
If physicians and licensed clinical psychologists become the only
providers allowed to administer direct biofeedback, it will rapidly
become a cost ineffective therapy. Furthermore, lack of state
licensure allows incompetent and dangerous biofeedback operations to
exist. If biofeedback does find its greatest use in medical as
opposed to psychiatric problems, it would seem that a biofeedback
therapist need not be a skilled psychotherapist. Certainly,
biofeedback as a medical and/or psychiatric therapy should be in
some way controlled by physicians, or, in the latter case, by
psychiatrists or clinical psychologists. These professionals need
not directly administer biofeedback, any more than orthopaedists
need directly administer physiotherapy. Biofeedback therapy can be
effectively administered if the biofeedback therapists are licensed.
This would create a health care specialist much like a registered
nurse or physical therapist. Biofeedback should be administered
only at the referral of a physician or licensed clinical psychologist. This would help ensure adequate pretreatment evaluation. A

licensed biofeedback therapist would have qualifications approximate
to a master's degree, with one to two years of special training.

Where should biofeedback be done? As with physiotherapy, for
example, biofeedback therapy can be performed either in a hospital
setting, that is, a biofeedback department, or in a freestanding
facility. In the former case, the department should have a physician director and should be staffed by licensed biofeedback therapists. Such a department would be open to referral from any
physician. The physician director should supervise quality control,
provide educational input, and communicate with the referring physicians in the event of inappropriate referrals. There specifically
need not be a biofeedback consult by such a director. Freestanding
biofeedback practices should use only licensed biofeedback therapists and should be allowed to accept only those cases referred by a
physician or licensed clinical psychologist. Such "free standing
offices" should also be strongly encouraged or even required to have
access to physician consultation and/or medical supervision.

Lacking any such licensure currently, one recommendation that
could be prudently made to a physician or psychologist intending to
begin to employ biofeedback is that he use only certified biofeedback therapists. This by no means guarantees competency and ethical
behavior, but certainly is at least a step in the right direction.

In the future, biofeedback could be practiced by a licensed
biofeedback therapist and/or an M.D., or licensed psychologist or
psychiatrist for psychiatric indications. Only a licensed biofeedback therapist would be allowed to call him- or herself by that
title.

CONCLUSION

In summary, then, this chapter has tried to offer a brief overview of the specific uses of biofeedback in medicine and a more
general discussion of biofeedback's current stance, both as a practical therapy and in the terms of certain theoretical conditions. A
few speculations as to the practical directions biofeedback should
take have been mentioned. In conclusion, biofeedback is emerging as
a viable and useful medical therapy which enjoys unusually low
toxicity. Biofeedback's relationship to clinical medicine is in the
formative stage, both theoretically and practically. This relationship will determine the future of biofeedback and who are to be its
practioners. Biofeedback, in a quiet way, represents a revolution
in medicine. It is indeed dated to hold that "cures" in the area of
health care are in the hands of an arcane brotherhood. Biofeedback
as a therapy allows the patient in a unique and especially rewarding
way to participate in the resolution of his or her problem.

[Editor's Note: In the opinion of one editor (WHR), this use of a
biofeedback technician who is unqualified by training or licensure
in a behavioral science discipline, such as psychology or psychiatry, by a professional without such training (i.e., medical special-
ties other than psychiatry) is proper, but unwise. A medical
license allows a physician to practice all of medicine, but it would
be an extremely foolish doctor who would try to perform an operation
such as cataract removal, heart surgery, etc. without thorough
training. Yet, state licensure does not distinguish between physicians in this way. Of course, leaving a patient alone in a room
connected to a biofeedback instrument with a relaxation tape or the
instructions "make the tone go down by warming your finger" is not
as risky as eye surgery. The risk in biofeedback therapy is far
more subtle. In many cases, patients need little help in mastering
the biofeedback task with symptomatic relief. There are also many
patients whose pathophysiology and/or personality disorders make
learning self-regulation extremely difficult. These people require
handling by an expert in psychodynamics and psychological therapy
for positive results. Otherwise, the patient assumes the blame for
failure with an increase in guilt and helplessness and the attendant
exacerbation in stress related symptoms and decrease in self-esteem
and motivational energy. Few malpractice suits are filed for these
problems and both patient and doctor are unaware of the part played
by biofeedback therapy in their genesis.]

DISCUSSION

     PARTICIPANT: I would just like to add a comment to the first
part of your talk when you took the example of the migraine person
who had two headaches a year and, therefore, the more traditional
medical treatment would be appropriate for cost benefits. My personal point of view would be that biofeedback or unstressing procedures or whatever this large category is called may, in fact, be
much more appropriate for those kinds of patients, especially if one
takes a long-time perspective. I realize that no prospective studies have been done using young people and then following for the
next 30 or 40 years to see what would happen if they had a more
prophylactic treatment or thinking. So my real suggestion is to
work just with those almost sub-clinical illnesses and teach those
people essentially health maintenance or health producing skills.

     GANS: We differ there. I respond to that and I respond to it
as a clinical strategy. You know, I don't know how many of you are
from Los Angeles. Everybody needs to get his act together and
everybody needs psychotherapy and I listen to Tony Grant every
chance I get in the car, O.K.? What I'm saying is, many of my
patients come to me and they have two migraines a year and they want
to know if I can fix it. And they are enjoying their surfing and
they are enjoying their work and they're enjoying their lives and

their stuff. We all may be laboring under undue levels of stress. The point is, they are not buying it, and they have a right to come in and say, "What have you got that is reasonably safe and expeditious to help me stop these headaches I get twice a year?" If they are likewise interested, and will recognize that they would like to cope differently with the kinds of things they view as stressors, that's one issue. If they're not, I don't try to push it on them.

PARTICIPANT: I don't have a question. I would like to say, I'm an internist in private practice near Los Angeles and I've been doing biofeedback training myself in a small way for about nine years and I agree wholeheartedly with everything you have said. Thank you.

REFERENCES

Aleo, S., & Nicassio, P. Autoregulation of duodenal ulcer disease. Proceedings of the Biofeedback Society of America, 1978, 278.

American Psychiatric Association Task Force on Biofeedback, (19), Washington, D. C.: American Psychiatric Association, 1981.

Baldwin, B. G., Benjamins, J. K. and Meyers, R., & Grant, C. W. EMG biofeedback with hyperactive children - a time series analysis. Proceedings of the Biofeedback Society of America, 1978, 184.

Blanchard, E. B. & Fahrion, S. Biofeedback and the modification of cardiovascular dysfunctions. Biofeedback Society of America Task Force Report, 1978.

Budzinski, T. & Stoyva, J. Biofeedback and temporomandibular joint syndrome. Journal of Dental Research, 1973, 52, 116-119.

Bueno-Miranda, F., Cerulli, M., & Shuster, M. Operant conditioning of colonic motility in irritable bowel syndrome (IBS). Journal of Gastroenterology, 1976, 20, 807.

Carlsson, S. G., Gale, E. N., & Ohman, A. Treatment of temporomandibular joint syndrome with biofeedback training. Journal of the American Dental Association, 1975, 91 (3), 602-605.

Cerulli, M. A., Nikoomanesh, P. & Shuster, M. M. Progress in biofeedback conditioning for fecal incontinence. Gastroenterology, 1976, 76, 742-746.

Cunningham, M. D., & Murphy, P. J. The effects of bilateral EEG biofeedback on verbal, visual spacial and creative skills in learning disabled male adolescents. Proceedings of the Biofeedback Society of America, 1978, 186.

Engel, B. T., Nikoomanesh, P., & Shuster, M. M. Operant conditioning of recto-sphincteric responses in the treatment of fecal incontinence. New England Journal of Medicine, 1974, 290, 646–649.

Engelhardt, L. Awareness and relaxation through biofeedback in public schools. Proceedings of the Biofeedback Society of America, 1978.

Fahrion, S. L. Task force study section update on biofeedback assisted treatment of essential hypertension. Biofeedback Society of America Task Force Addendum, 1979.

Finley, William W. Demonstration of EMG reward system for biofeedback work with children. Proceedings of the Biofeedback Society of America, 1979, 254.

Furman, S. Intestinal biofeedback in functional diarrhea, a preliminary report. Journal of Behavioral Therapy and Experimental Psychiatry, 1973, 4, 317–321.

Gerber, L. Biofeedback for patients with Raynaud's phenomenon. Journal of the American Medical Association, 1979, 242 (6), 509–510.

Gorman, P. Cephalic influences on human gastric acid secretion and their voluntary control through biofeedback training. Dissertation Abstracts International, 1976, 36 (12–B, Pt 1), 6413.

Greenspan, K., & Lawrence, R. The role of biofeedback in arterial occlusive disease. Journal of Surgical Research, 1980.

Gregg, R. H. The use of biofeedback in labor, OB-GYN Observer, June, July 1975.

Hartman, C. H. The response of anginal pain to hand warming. Biofeedback and self-regulation, 1979, 4(4), 355–357.

Hiebert, B., & Fitzsimmons, G. W. A comparison of EMG feedback and alternative anxiety treatment program. Proceedings of the Biofeedback Society of America, 1979, 22–25.

Hughes, R., & Collins, N. Group instruction and relaxation training with nursery school children. Proceedings of the Biofeedback Society of America, 1978, 147.

Jankel, W. R. EMG feedback in spasmodic torticollis. Proceedings of the Biofeedback Society of America, 1978, 124.

Jeffery, T. B. The effects of operant conditioning and electromyographic biofeedback on the relaxed behavior of hyperkinetic children. Proceedings of the Biofeedback Society of America, 1978, 192.

Jensen, J. S., & Stoffer, G. R. The treatment of essential blepharospasm. Paper presented at the Biofeedback Society of America, 1978.

Kay, M., Shiverly, M., & Kilkenny, J. Training sensorimotor
     rhythm in developmentally disabled children through EEG
     biofeedback. Proceedings of the Biofeedback Society of
     America, 1978, 195.

Koheil, R., Mandel, A., & Iles, G. Joint position training for
     hyperextension of the knee in stroke patients,
     preliminary results. Proceedings of the Biofeedback
     Society of America, 1979, 119-122.

Lubar, J. et al. EEG feedback training in epileptics
     controlled multidimensional studies. Progress Report,
     Proceedings of the Biofeedback Society of America, 1979,
     127-130.

Mandel, A. R. & Sharp, E. Biofeedback versus conditional
     physiotherapy as a means of improving head control in
     children with cerebral palsy. Proceedings of the
     Biofeedback Society of America, 1979, 131-134.

Marcus, N. & Legin, G. Clinical applications of biofeedback:
     Implications for psychiatry. Journal Hospital and
     Community Psychiatry Society, 1977, 28(1), 21-25.

Marlatt, A. G., Rose, R. R., Pagano, R. R., & Marques, J. K.
     Effects of meditation and relaxation training on alcohol
     use in male social drinkers. Proceedings of the
     Biofeedback Society of America, 1978, 169.

Matulich, W. J., Rugh, J. D., & Perlis, D. B. A comparison
     of group and individual EMG feedback for tension
     headaches. Proceedings of the Biofeedback Society of
     America, 1978, 58.

McCrady, A. V., Tan, S. D., Crane, R., & Fine, T.,
     Biochemical correlates of biofeedback in essential
     hypertension. Citation Paper, Proceedings of the
     Biofeedback Society of America, 1979, 79.

Patmon, R., & Murphy, P. J. Differential treatment efficacy
     of EEG and EMG feedback for hyperactive adolescents.
     Proceedings of the Biofeedback Society of America, 1978,
     179.

Reinking, R. P. Biofeedback as an adjunct to alcoholism
     treatment. Proceedings of the Biofeedback Society of
     America, 1978, 172.

Rickles, W. H. Biofeedback, therapy, and transitional pheno-
     mena in therapy of psychosomatic/narcissistic disorders.
     Psychiatric Annals, 1981, 11(3), 23-41.

Rubow, R., & Netsell, R. EMG biofeedback rehabilitation in
     facial paralysis, a ten year follow-up of a case study.
     Proceedings of the Biofeedback Society of America, 1979,
     139.

Sandweiss, J., Diamond, S., & Adler, C. Symposium on
     biofeedback and vascular headache. Presented at the
     Biofeedback Society of America Convention, 1982.

Sargent, J. G., Greene, E. E., & Walters, D. E. Biofeedback
    in migraine headaches. Psychosomatic Medicine, 1973,
    35(2), 129-135.
Sedlacek, K. EMG, GSR, and thermal biofeedback in the treat-
    ment of hypertension. Biofeedback and Self-Regulation,
    1976, 1(3), 311-312.
Sedlacek, K. Biofeedback for Raynaud's disease.
    Psychosomatics, 1979, 20(8), 535-541.
Sedlacek, K. & Heczey, M. A specific biofeedback training
    for dysmenorrhea. Proceedings of the Biofeedback
    Society of America, 1977.
Shabsin, H. S., Bahler, W., & Lubar, J. F. A comparison of
    twelve to fifteen Hz Rolandic Activity (SMR) during eyes
    open and eyes closed conditions and its occurence with
    occipital alpha. Proceedings of the Biofeedback Society
    of America, 1978, 165.
Shavoy, G., Williams, R. R., & Johnson, G. EMG biofeedback
    assisted catecholamine suppression during response to
    individual stress. Proceedings of the Biofeedback
    Society of Michigan, State Meeting, 1979.
Tubbs, W., & Carnahan, C. Clinical biofeedback for primary
    dysmenorrhea: Pilot study. Biofeedback and Self-
    Regulation, 1976, 1(3), 323.
Werbach, M., & Sandweiss, J. H. Peripheral temperatures in
    migrainers undergoing relaxation training. Headache,
    1978, 18(4), 211-214.

BIOFEEDBACK AND RAYNAUD'S DIATHESIS

Robert N. Grove

Clinical Psychophysiology, Veteran's Hospital
Sepulveda, California
UCLA School of Medicine
Los Angeles, California

and

Muriel T. Belanger

Psychology Department
Laval University
Quebec, Canada

During routine examinations, the health professional is likely
to encounter patients who complain of cold hands. Very few patients,
however, exhibit the severe vasospastic episodes characteristic of
Raynaud's diathesis. Nevertheless, some Raynaud's patients remain
unaware of the unusual nature of their symptoms until severe organic
changes become apparent. Health professionals, capable of differen-
tially diagnosing Raynaud's diathesis during its early stages, may
be able to stabilize or abolish these early symptoms using traditional medicine and biobehavioral techniques such as biofeedback.

The goal of this chapter is to aid the professional in the
diagnosis and treatment of this disorder. The first part of the
chapter reviews the etiology, mechanisms and differential diagnosis
of Raynaud's diathesis. That section concludes with a psychophysiological comparison of Raynaud's patients with healthy volunteers
conducted in our laboratory. The second part reviews traditional
treatments, the use of biofeedback in Raynaud's diathesis, and
concludes with case studies of a new biofeedback procedure, localized cold inoculation training, in patients with Raynaud's disease
or with Raynaud's phenomenon secondary to scleroderma.

193

PART I: DIAGNOSIS OF RAYNAUD'S DIATHESIS: CLINICAL, PSYCHOLOGICAL
          AND PSYCHOPHYSIOLOGICAL CONSIDERATIONS

RAYNAUD'S DISEASE AND RAYNAUD'S PHENOMENON

     Raynaud's disease/phenomenon is a peripheral thermoregulatory
disorder of diverse etiologies. It is characterized by episodes of
extreme cooling of the hands, feet or parts of the face and tongue
(Spittell, 1974). The accepted immediate cause for these episodes
is either low environmental temperatures and/or emotional stress
(Mittleman & Wolff, 1943; Blair et al., 1951; Graham, 1955, 1974;
Graham et al., 1958). During a prolonged vasospastic episode, the
skin color of the affected area blanches, then turns cyanotic and
finally red during remission. An attack is often accompanied by a
sensation of tingling or pain. In severe cases, Raynaud's disease/
phenomenon may result in severe pain in the digits, ulcer formation,
and even gangrene. Autoamputation of the fingers is not uncommon.
When episodic peripheral vasospasm is seen independently of any
other disorder, it is diagnosed as Raynaud's disease. When it is
observed with a variety of related disorders, it is diagnosed as
Raynaud's phenomenon. Raynaud's phenomenon is an associated symptom
in many post-traumatic occupational diseases (e.g., pneumatic hammer
disease, typist's fingers), occlusive arterial diseases (e.g.,
arteriosclerosis obliterans), toxic substance syndromes (e.g., heavy
metal poisoning, ergot intoxication) and diverse diseases such as
rheumatoid arthritis, lupus erythematosus, and scleroderma
(Spittell, 1974; Velayos et al., 1971; Birostingl, 1971; Fries,
1967). Migraine headache has been observed in 14% of Raynaud's
patients and hypertension in 9% (Gifford and Hines, 1957).

     This presentation will focus upon two types of peripheral
vasoregulatory disorders: Raynaud's disease and Raynaud's phenomenon associated with scleroderma.

Raynaud's Disease

     The diagnosis of "pure" Raynaud's disease is dependent upon (a)
negative findings in tests for associated diseases, and (b) the continued presence of idiopathic, episodic vasospasms spanning at least
two years (Spittell, 1974). A number of theories have emerged to
explain the symptoms. Current research generally supports the
theory of excessive sympathetic discharge as the immediate cause of
Raynaud's disease, although in a small minority of cases (four of 66
patients) abnormal clumping of red blood cells or precipitation of
globulin may be directly involved (DeTakato & Fowler, 1962;
Pringle et al., 1965). Peacock (1959) found an elevated catecholamine level in blood taken from the wrist of patients with Raynaud's
disease, suggesting a continuous sympathetic vasoconstrictor
hyperactivity. This finding could not be replicated in either
Raynaud's disease patients (Kontos & Wasserman, 1969) or in

patients with scleroderma-associated Raynaud's phenomenon (Sapira et al., 1972).

An alternative theory, receptor hypersensitivity in vascular smooth muscle, was put forward by Jamieson, Ludbrook and Wilson (1971). Here, the vasoconstrictive alpha-receptors are believed to be hyper-responsive to normal levels of circulating catecholamines. However, other investigators have failed to find either increased reflex sympathetic vasoconstriction to cold stimuli (Downey & Frewin, 1973), or an increased sensitivity to intravenous norepinephrine (Mendlowitz & Naftchi, 1959). On the other hand, some, although not all, patients have been found to exhibit an increased digital sympathetic vasomotor tone (Mendlowitz & Naftchi, 1959).

The origin and mechanisms involved in the triggering and maintenance of these episodes in Raynaud's disease remains unresolved. A controversy exists as to whether a purely functional vasospasm characterizing Raynaud's disease is in fact an early indicator of impending organic vascular disease. If Raynaud's disease exists for two years without the appearance of any associated disease, 95% of patients do not go on to develop any such secondary disease (Gifford & Hines, 1957). It is on this basis that the clinician waits at least two years before concluding that the patient has "pure" Raynaud's disease. In advanced cases of Raynaud's disease, it is common to observe a thickening of the digital capillaries concurrent with frequent, severe attacks. Ulceration and scarring may also occasionally be found.

In a recent review, Coffman and Davies (1975) hypothesized that the critical factor in the early stages of Raynaud's disease may be the chronically reduced blood flow to the extremities caused largely by heightened sympathetic vasomotor tone. An external cold-stimulus should produce the same quantity of vasoconstriction as is observed in normal subjects; however, the already-reduced baseline digital blood flow (and pressure), hypothesized to exist in Raynaud's patients, are presumed to establish conditions wherein the additional vasoconstriction could reduce flow below some critical value, thus inducing ischemia. In mild Raynaud's disease, this ischemia is believed to sensitize further the digital vessels to a transient state of increased vascular tone, further reducing blood flow. As the disease progresses, secondary thickening of the vascular walls would mask or limit the influence of increased tone. By this formulation, then, reduced blood flow is the precipitating factor.

While Raynaud's disease appears to be relatively easily understood at a conceptual level, its individual clinical manifestations are often unpredictable. Large-scale clinical studies (Velayos et al., 1971) fail to describe adequately the individual course of the disease, either before, during, or following treatment.

Raynaud's episodes are typically localized to specific fingers or toes. A clinical feature of Raynaud's disease (and phenomenon) is that some fingers and toes are more affected than others. Furthermore, it is not uncommon for the pattern of affected fingers and toes to change over time. Treatment outcome studies often fail to document changes in more than one finger. It is not known from such single site temperature studies whether (a) other digits are equally affected by the disorder, or (b) whether the treatment effect may have coincided with a spontaneous shift in the pattern of digits affected away from the targeted finger or toe.

Raynaud's Phenomenon

Raynaud's phenomenon is characterized by the presence of an associated disease which influences the CNS, the immune system, and/or the viscera. Ongoing research is exploring the possibility that peripheral vasospasms may be accompanied by blood flow restrictions in the kidney and lung, at least for some disorders.

Renal vasospastic episodes. Cannon (1975) supplied a convincing demonstration that Raynaud's phenomenon could affect the vasculature of the viscera. By using a radioactive xenon washout technique, he determined that there was significant renal arteriolar vasospasm and significant reductions in renal blood flow in some subjects at a time when Raynaud's phenomenon was occurring in the hands. More recently, Kovalchik et al. (1978) demonstrated that there is an elevation of renin, a renal hormone, in response to cold exposure in subjects who had exhibited histologic evidence of sclerodermatous involvement in the renal vasculature. Presumably, renin was released in response to a reduction in renal blood flow during cold exposure, a phenomenon not found in normal subjects during exposure to a cold challenge.

Pulmonary vasospastic episodes. Clements and Furst tested several scleroderma patients using radioactive Krypton coupled with lung scanning to assess pulmonary blood flow dysregulation (1980, personal communication). Their results show significant reductions in blood volume in the lungs during exposure of the hands to cold. Davis et al. (1979) found similar results for pulmonary flow in response to stressors. Together, these studies provide strong support for visceral involvement induced by a brief cold stress to the extremities.

Herzog et al. (1980) found a high incidence of visceral abnormalities in 39 scleroderma patients followed in the UCLA Rheumatology Clinic. More than 95% of the 39 patients also had Raynaud's phenomenon in the hands. The authors speculate that Raynaud's phenomenon in the extremities may be associated with vasospasm and damage to the viscera. However, the question of whether cold-induced vasospasm causes or precipitates sclerodermatous structural

changes within the viscera remains as yet unanswered. Rigorous clinical research remains to be conducted to verify whether or not
peripheral Raynaud's phenomenon is an early precursor of more
serious heart, lung, and renal disorders.

Psychological Variables in Raynaud's Diathesis

Except for a handful of clinical reports and the small group
studies mentioned below, little is known about the precise psychological makeup of Raynaud's patients. Emotion (Mittlemann & Wolff,
1939, 1943) is likely to elicit a vasospastic episode. The
available clinical reports favor the hypothesis that Raynaud's phenomenon is frequently associated with either hostility or anxiety in
the face of emotional stimuli (Mittlemann & Wolff, 1943).

D. T. Graham (1955) found that vasospastic episodes in four
Raynaud's patients were always associated with signs or expressions
of hostility. Mufson (1944, 1953) suggests that these patients are
likely to be chronically anxious because of their excessive sensitivity to actual or perceived threats of death, resentment or loss
of a loved one. After successfully treating three Raynaud's
patients with psychoanalytic therapy, Millet, Lief and Mittlemann
(1953) concluded that vasospastic attacks resembled anxiety attacks
and added that these patients are likely to be both hysterical and
obsessive-compulsive in managing their guilt feelings.

This conclusion was later modified by Millet (1956). He speculated that the vasospastic episodes should probably not be considered a pure conversion reaction. Instead, he proposed that
Raynaud's disease was initially a conditioned vasomotor response to
"fear of the contact with death," anticipated death, or rejection of
a loved one. This extreme response was seen to be self-sustaining.
The patients' perceived guilt for having these fears would be properly punished by subsequent attacks.

However, it is premature to conclude that a specific personality configuration can be identified for Raynaud's patients, even if
one exists. The multiple causes of the diathesis and the available
evidence suggest only that the disorder may be linked in some way to
psychological as well as pathophysiological factors. Hostility and
anxiety may indeed be involved in this disorder, but it is not
apparent why non-Raynaud's patients fail to experience similar
extreme vasospastic episodes under the same conditions. It is
possible that patients with Raynaud's disease and Raynaud's phenomenon simply have a more reactive vasoconstrictor response than other
patients. On the other hand, we are dealing with patients who are
experiencing chronic intermittent pain and functional immobility.
In our laboratory, we often observe clinically relevant long-term
behavioral changes such as those found for other chronic pain
patients (e.g., Fordyce 1975; Sternbach, 1974). It is common to

observe depression, anxiety, and hostility in such patients, but it
is not clear whether such factors are directly involved in the precipitation or maintenance of a particular disorder.

EXPERIMENT I: PSYCHOPHYSIOLOGICAL ASSESSMENT OF RAYNAUD'S DIATHESIS

The major goal of this experiment was to assess peripheral
temperature and peripheral blood flow in Raynaud's patients during
exposure to stressful emotional and cold stimuli. The psychophysiological stress profile consisted of the following tests: stabilization period (10 minutes) random; orienting response tones (22
minutes); mental arithmetic (10 minutes); rest period (5 minutes);
cold challenge (20 minutes); and rest period (5 minutes). Pulse
wave amplitudes of the right and left index fingers were measured
and recorded.

Fifteen patients with Raynaud's diathesis and 15 non-Raynaud's
normal controls were given the psychophysiological stress profile.
The age of the Raynaud's patients ranged from 33 to 72 years old.
There were 14 females and one male. The patient pool consisted of
three "pure" Raynaud's disease subjects and 12 patients with
Raynaud's phenomenon secondary to progressive systemic sclerosis.
Duration of disease ranged from three years to 20 years.

There were 15 non-Raynaud's healthy control subjects (three
males, 12 females) ranging in age from 23 to 54 years.

Apparatus

The experimental room of the Clinical Psychophysiology
Service, VA Medical Center, Sepulveda, served as the locale for the
psychophysiological stress test. The 16' x 10' x 10' room was
acoustically shielded and isolated from the programming apparatus
located in the adjacent room. During the experimental sessions, a
table lamp with a shaded 75-watt bulb served as the sole source of
illumination.

The subject was seated in an acoustically-baffled, egg-shaped
fiberglass "stereo lounger" chair, modified for physiological
recording. The chair was foam-padded and featured a head rest and
foam-padded arm rests. The seat was adjusted so that the arms were
always resting at the level of the heart, thus standardizing
peripheral pulse recording. The cold plate was recessed into the
left arm of the chair. The feet were elevated on a stool.

The temperature thermistors (Yellow Springs Instruments
Series 700 termilinear probe No. 709, 3/8" diameter) had a 1.1
second time constant. Pulse wave amplitude (PWA) was monitored by a
stick-on infrared LED-phototransistor sensor attached to the finger

pad of the middle digit. It had a frequency response range of 0.5
Hz to 10.0 Hz (Coulbourn Instruments).

A thermoelectric cold plate (Thermoelectrics, Model TCP-2)
with a 3" diameter top plate was used for the cold challenge test.
Temperature of the cold plate was regulated with a Bio-Feedback
Technology, Inc., BFT-301, feedback thermometer. The thermistor was
attached directly to the cold plate and its temperature was
controlled manually via a rheostat accessible to the experimenter in
the control room.

The Raynaud's patients were selected from the patient pool of
the UCLA Rheumatology Division. Non-Raynaud's controls were
recruited from hospital staff, university students, and friends of
patients. Patients were selected only if (1) they had demonstrated
Raynaud's phenomenon to one of the referring physicians or
investigators, and (2) they met the criteria for primary Raynaud's
disease or for Raynaud's phenomenon associated with scleroderma.

"Pure" Raynaud's patients demonstrated all of the following
criteria: (1) Raynaud's phenomenon; (2) absence of gangrenous
lesions; (3) absence of any systemic disease that might account for
the occurrence of Raynaud's phenomenon; and (4) duration of
Raynaud's phenomenon for a minimum of two years without appearance
of any connective tissue disorders.

All scleroderma patients were required to demonstrate a
Raynaud's episode (Raynaud's vasospasm) in the presence of one of
the investigators. The observed vasospasm could either be spontaneous or induced by a cold pressor test (i.e., a hand or foot held
in ice water for 2 to 5 minutes).

The diagnosis for scleroderma required the presence of one or
two minor criteria:

(1) <u>Major</u>: Taut or hidebound skin involving the skin of
the face and fingers.

(2) <u>Minor</u>: (a) Sclerodactyly (tight skin on fingers)

(b) Digital pitting scars (on fingers)

(c) Interstitial fibrosis (on chest x-ray)

(d) Colonic pseudosacculation (on barium
enema)

These criteria represent modifications of previously published
criteria which have been utilized to conform to the preliminary

diagnosis for scleroderma as proposed by the American Rheumatism
Association (Fries & Medsgar, 1978).

Procedure

Upon arrival at the Clinical Psychophysiology Service,
patients were asked to read and sign the informed consent forms, a
medical history was taken, and the psychophysiological test battery
was administered. Patients were then requested to fill out the
Symptom Daily Log Charts for one week. Normal controls were only
requested to sign informed consent forms and undergo the psychophysiological test battery. They were not asked to fill out the
charts.

Informed consent forms were read and signed by patients. A
brief explanation of the testing procedure was given. A review of
the medical history of the patient and of his family was taken.
Detailed information was sought regarding Raynaud's vasospastic
attacks and its associated disorder.

Finger temperature was monitored by thermistors placed on
the dorsal surface of the index fingers, and pulse wave amplitude
(PWA) was measured by placing Coulbourn Instruments photoplethysmographic transducers on the ventral surface of the middle fingers
over the finger pad. Signals from these sensors were amplified on
an 8-channel, Beckman Type RM Dynagraph polygraph. These same
signals were fed to analog-to-digital converters (Coulbourn
Instruments), then to a printer. Digital data was key-boarded into
an Apple II computer program for conversion to degrees Centigrade
and millivolts (PWA).

The psychophysiological stress battery consisted of the
following:

(a) <u>Rest I</u>: Stabilization (10 minutes)

The patient was requested to rest quietly for 10
minutes for stabilization of physiology.

(b) <u>Orienting Response</u>: (22 minutes)

This test evaluates the degree of responsiveness, in
terms of rise and fall of temperature and amount of vasoconstriction
and vasodilitation, to a series of tones. The subject was asked to
sit quietly while a tape of white noise tones was presented. A
series of 30 tones (duration: 40 milliseconds), consisting of 60
dbs, 70 dbs, 80 dbs, 90 dbs, and 100 dbs, was presented at variable
intervals (average = 30 seconds) for a period of 22 minutes.

(c) Mental Arithmetic

This test assessed stress responses during a high demand task requiring continuous concentration.

The 10 minute test was divided into two segments: addition and subtraction. The first part involved the oral presentation of three sets of two-digit numbers for summation. The final five minute segment of the test consisted of subtracting sevens, starting from 801, until either 0 was reached or time was up. The subject was required to give verbally the correct solution as rapidly as possible. The subtest had been found to be a reliable means of eliciting considerable psychological stress (Cohen et al., 1978).

(d) Rest II (5 minutes)

The subject was requested to rest quietly for five minutes so that his physiology could once again stabilize.

(e) Cold Challenge (20 minutes)

This test was done to evaluate the extent of physiological responses (vasoconstriction/dilitation and temperature rise/drop) during discrete controlled temperature decreases.

The patient's left palm was placed on a thermoelectric cold plate. The initial plate temperature was $29.4^{\circ}C$ ($85^{\circ}F$), $23.9^{\circ}C$ ($75^{\circ}F$), OFF 1 (i.e., thermoelectric plate was turned off and allowed to return to room temperature for two minutes), $18.3^{\circ}C$ ($65^{\circ}F$), OFF 2, $12.8^{\circ}C$ ($55^{\circ}F$), OFF 3, $7.2^{\circ}C$ ($45^{\circ}F$), OFF 4, $7.2^{\circ}C$ ($45^{\circ}F$). Physiological recording commenced only when the desired temperature of the cold plate was reached (e.g., $18.3^{\circ} \pm 1.0^{\circ}C$). The plate temperature during the OFF segments returned to $29.4^{\circ}C$.

(f) Rest III (5 minutes)

The subject was instructed to rest quietly for a final five minutes of physiological recording. Particular attention was given during this period to the extent of recovery (i.e., compared to Rest I) of the subject from the cold stimulus.

Data Analysis

The major question posed in this experiment was whether or not there are any diagnostically relevant differences between the Raynaud's patients and the non-Raynaud's healthy control subjects in their physiological responses to stress. Subtest scores were examined to assess which components were the most sensitive to physiological changes. A comparison was made between the subtest physiological responses of patients with scleroderma (n = 12) and those with "pure" Raynaud's disease (n = 3).

Raynaud's Group vs. Control Group: Mean Differences. The profile data were split into nine components: stabilization (10
minutes), early orienting response (11 minutes), late orienting
response (11 minutes), early mental arithmetic (5 minutes), late
mental (5 minutes), rest (5 minutes), early cold (29.4°C, 23.9°C,
18.3°C), late cold (12.8°C, 7.2°C, 7.2°C), and rest (5 minutes).
Dividing each of the three tasks into early and late halves permitted a statistical comparison of the stability of the response
pattern within tasks. The means of each of the nine components of
each hand were then calculated, as well as the lowest and the
highest score of each component.

1. Finger Temperature Profiles

A three-way analysis of variance for repeated measures on two
factors was conducted for the absolute left and right hand finger
temperatures in degrees centigrade. This analysis was statistically
significant for the between-subjects factor for group membership (df
= 1, 359, F = 0.94, P $\leq$ .01). No other main effect or interactions
were significant. Thus, the Raynaud's group differed from the
control group across tasks and across hands (left and right).

Because the overall F-value was significant, multiple t-test
comparisons between task means for the cold-exposed left hands of
two groups were permissible. Interestingly, multiple t-tests between the overall group mean differences collapsed across tasks for
the left hand yielded no significant differences (t = 0.91, 28 df,
p $\leq$ 0.85). As a group, Raynaud's patients showed a mean-left-hand
across session temperature of 30.00 + 2.14°C, compared to 30.70 +
2.21°C for controls. Next, the across-session means for the 12
scleroderma patients were analyzed separately. This scleroderma
subgroup mean of 29.85 + 2.38°C was lower than either the mean of
the controls or the mean temperature of the three Raynaud's disease
patients (30.60 + 0.61o$_C$). However, this difference was not statistically significant at the p =$\leq$.05 level (t = 0.98, 25 df, p $\leq$
0.15).

The group membership difference is also reflected in Table 2,
which shows the mean right- and left-hand temperatures for both
groups across tasks. Raynaud's patients generally showed lower temperatures across tasks than controls. During the Rest 1, the left-
hand temperature of the Raynaud's group, for example, was 30.29 +
2.54°C (column 1, row 1), while the control group's temperature was
31.07 + 2.79°C.

Three differences distinguish the pattern of temperature
responses of the control and experimental groups:

(a) For the Raynaud's group, mean left-hand temperature declined across tasks from 30.28 to 29.01°C. For controls, mean temperature held rather constant (31.12°C) across tasks.

(b) The groups also differed on the tasks which yielded the largest mean temperature decrements. For the Raynaud's group, the largest mean drop occurred during the last rest (29.01°C ± 2.38°C), followed by late cold challenge (29.56°C ± 1.99°C), then early cold challenge (30.00°C ± 2.07°C). For the control group, the largest mean decrement occurred during late MA (30.15°C 2.05°C), and early MA (30.40°C ± 2.54°C), then to late cold challenge (30.47°C ± 2.26°C).

(c) The early and late cold challenge tasks and the post-cold recovery period showed the greatest group mean differences. During cold challenge, the Raynaud's group showed a mean drop of more than 1°C (from 30.13°C pre-cold to 29.01°C post-cold), while control means rose almost 0.5°C (from 30.69°C to 31.12°C). These differences suggest that, in addition to being more sensitive to cold, Raynaud's patients lack the ability to recover rapidly from cold (see Table 1).

Visual inspection of the right-hand temperature changes reveal an identical pattern of differences between the Raynaud's group and the control group. The right-hand temperatures dropped in response to a graded cold challenge to the left hand. This contralateral temperature shift cannot be due to local cooling, but must be mediated by central changes in autonomic vasomotor reactivity.

Table 2 shows the mean temperatures and standard deviations of the experimental group divided into the scleroderma and Raynaud's disease subgroups. It is remarkable that the scleroderma patients reacted to the cold challenge in almost the same manner as the control group, while the Raynaud's subgroup experienced a drop of 3.0°C in the left hand and almost 2.5°C in the right hand (Table 2).

2.   Finger Pulse Amplitude Profiles

Absolute finger peak pulse amplitudes were calculated from the gain factor necessary to maintain a standard pulse signal by infrared reflectance photoplethysmography of the middle finger. This signal was quantified through a voltage peak detector coupled to a cumulating-resetting integrator and expressed as the product of the signal gain factor times the resetting constant factor in millivolt seconds. A three-way analysis of variance for repeated measures on two factors (group membership and left- or right-hand responses) yielded two statistically significant effects ($P \leq .10$).

The variance ratios were statistically significant for both

Table 1

	Rest	Early OR	Late OR	Early MA	Late MA	Rest	Early C	Late C	Rest
LEFT HAND -- TEMPERATURE °C									
Raynaud's Diathesis									
X̄	3.287	3.37	30.21	30.09	30.15	30.13	30.00	29.56	29.01
SD	± 2.54	± 2.11	± 2.24	± 2.34	± 2.36	± 2.30	± 2.07	± 1.99	± 2.38
Control									
X̄	31.07	31.17	30.74	30.40	30.15	30.69	30.79	30.47	31.12
SD	± 2.79	± 2.53	± 2.86	± 2.54	± 2.05	± 2.21	± 2.41	± 2.26	± 3.06
RIGHT HAND -- TEMPERATURE °C									
Raynaud's Diathesis									
X̄	31.65	31.33	31.26	31.29	31.48	31.68	31.05	30.74	30.90
SD	± 2.30	± 2.82	± 2.87	± 2.54	± 2.38	± 2.47	± 2.54	± 2.33	± 2.54
Control									
X̄	31.95	31.95	31.69	31.41	31.27	31.91	31.82	31.53	32.11
SD	± 1.36	± 2.00	± 2.60	± 1.96	± 1.58	± 1.95	± 2.09	± 2.32	± 2.04

Legend: Rest = Stabilization; Early OR and Late OR = Orienting Response with random tone presentations (60-100dB); Early MA = Mental Arithmetic (addition); Late MA = Mental Arithmetic (subtraction); Rest; Early C = Cold Challenge (29.4°C, 23.9°C, 18.3°C); Late C = Cold Challenge (12.8°C, 7.2°C, 7.2°C); Rest

group membership (df = 1, 28, F = 26.44, P ≤ 0.005) and the hand measured (df = 1, 28, F = 8.24, P ≤ 0.10). These results may be clarified by post-hoc multiple t-test comparisons of pulse amplitude data from left hand, which was generally more responsive to the left-palmar cold stimulus. When collapsed across all tasks, the Raynaud's group exhibited somewhat greater left-hand vasoconstriction (9.54 ± 8.46 mV-sec) than the healthy control group (22.67 ± 10.5 mV-sec) (df = 28, t = 1.38, P = 0.08). This group difference trend appears to be due to the predominance of scleroderma patients in the experimental group.

As shown in Table 3, the twelve scleroderma patients, as a group, exhibited significantly greater vasoconstriction (6.00 ± 4.10 mV-sec) across tasks than the three Raynaud's disease patients as a group (23.72 ± 5.61 mV-sec) (t = 1.96, 25 df, P< 0.05).

Group difference deviations in individual absolute pulse amplitudes (mV-sec) were so large that an evaluation of the tasks which most clearly distinguished between Raynaud's patients and controls were washed out by extreme between-subjects variability. However, by transforming the individual absolute pulse amplitudes to individual range-corrected scores (see Cohen, McArthur and Rickles, 1978), it was possible to identify task specific changes relative to the individual's overall vasomotor responsivity across an entire session. Range-corrected scores were computed by first identifying the highest (100%) and lowest (0%) absolute one minute peak pulse wave amplitude scores (in millivolt-seconds) across each subject's entire session. Each absolute task score was then subtracted from the lowest session score (0%), and the difference was divided by the difference between the highest (100%) and the lowest (0%) session scores. An individualized, range corrected score (in percent of session range) was thus computed for each task for each subject. These individualized task-specific, range corrected percents were summed across groups and used to calculate group mean scores and deviations, as shown in Table 3.

Relative pulse amplitudes of the 12 scleroderma patients were first analyzed separately from the three Raynaud's disease patients (See Table 4). When averaged across all tasks, the relative amplitude for the scleroderma group was 32.35 ± 9.18%, and, for the Raynaud's disease group, 38.77 ± 7.00%. The control group averaged 37 ± 10.31% of range across all tasks. There were no statistically meaningful differences between groups. Thus, when individual differences in absolute pulse amplitudes are adjusted for by the range correction procedure, overall range-corrected scores fail to uncover any discernible vasomotor pattern differences between the experimental and control groups, and between the scleroderma and Raynaud's disease patients. All of our subjects, when grouped and averaged, tended to demonstrate mild constriction and large variability (32.35 to 38.77%) averaged across all tasks.

Table 2

	Rest	Early OR	Late OR	Early MA	Late MA	Rest	Early C	Late C	Rest
LEFT HAND -- TEMPERATURE °C									
Scleroderma (n = 12)									
X̄	29.87	30.1	29.85	30.0	29.85	29.89	30.1	29.72	29.48
SD	± 2.7	± 2.28	± 2.4	± 2.25	± 2.59	± 2.54	± 2.27	± 2.24	± 2.29
Raynaud's Disease (n = 3)									
X̄	31.94	31.45	31.64	31.44	31.33	31.09	29.6	28.91	28.05
SD	± 0.98	± 0.96	± 0.79	± 0.84	± 0.5	± 0.83	± 0.91	± 0.48	± 0.65
RIGHT HAND -- TEMPERATURE °C									
Scleroderma (n = 12)									
X̄	31.53	31.15	30.98	31.03	31.16	31.49	31.2	31.04	31.09
SD	± 2.47	± 3.04	± 3.09	± 2.74	± 2.59	± 2.69	± 2.75	± 2.52	± 2.57
Raynaud's Disease (n = 3)									
X̄	32.13	32.04	32.39	32.3	32.75	32.42	30.48	29.54	30.24
SD	± 1.73	± 1.75	± 1.6	± 1.28	± 0.65	± 1.33	± 1.23	± 1.13	± 1.23

Legend: See Legend of Table 1 for explanation of tasks.

Table 3

	Rest	Early OR	Late OR	Early MA	Late MA	Rest	Early C	Late C	Rest
LEFT HAND -- PULSE WAVE AMPLITUDE (mV-S)									
Scleroderma (n = 12)									
X̄	8.28	5.92	4.94	5.05	5.65	7.64	5.6	4.26	5.93
SD	± 8.22	± 4.64	± 3.96	± 4.44	± 3.66	± 7.05	± 4.0	± 2.14	± 4.86
Raynaud's Disease (n = 3)									
X̄	27.26	23.81	27.63	21.25	19.02	29.32	14.6	14.76	35.8
SD	± 14.56	± 11.5	± 12.53	± 4.34	± 2.35	± 9.02	± 5.99	± 8.93	± 19.55
RIGHT HAND -- PULSE WAVE AMPLITUDE (mV-S)									
Scleroderma (n = 12)									
X̄	8.06	.83	8.13	7.46	7.72	8.96	8.87	7.72	9.17
SD	± 7.69	± 8.41	± 8.6	± 8.04	± 8.56	± 9.95	± 9.58	± 8.07	± 8.49
Raynaud's Disease (n = 3)									
X̄	41.19	35.7	32.03	24.48	25.36	32.47	23.14	22.8	30.78
SD	± 9.01	± 15.14	± 6.2	± 6.06	± 5.9	± 8.14	± 6.52	± 8.03	± 18.56

Legend: See Legend of Table 1 for explanation of tasks.

Table 3 shows the mean range-corrected pulse amplitudes and standard deviations for the experimental and control groups across tasks. In interpreting the data in Table 3, it is important to remember that these tabularized scores represent the <u>relative</u> degree of constriction (approaching 0%) or dilation (approaching 100%) for an individual across a task, relative to his highest and lowest one minute responses within that session. These are <u>not</u> absolute values of capillary bed vasomotor response.

For the left hand PWA (upper rows, Table 3), the Raynaud's group during the first rest demonstrated marked relative vaso-constriction (38.9 ± 37.4% of range) accompanied by enormous variability. During the same rest, the control group mean relative range was 57.0 ± 20.0%. Thus, as a group, Raynaud's patients entered the stress test with greater mean vasoconstriction, and showed greater individual variability as indexed by the standard deviation of left-hand resting ranges.

Across tasks, the trend in relative vasoconstriction is just the opposite of that found for temperature. Whereas mean tem-peratures dropped markedly across tasks for the Raynaud's group but not controls (see Table 3), the opposite occurred for range-corrected PWA. Here the relative mean PWA's for the Raynaud's group showed little variation across tasks (from 38.9% on the first rest to 37.4% on the last rest), while for the control group, relative PWA's dropped from 57.0% to 42.3% from Rest 1 to final rest.

The groups also differed on the selection of tasks which yielded the largest left-hand mean relative vasoconstriction scores. Raynaud's patients vasoconstricted mostly to cold, while controls vasoconstricted mostly to a cognitive stressor. For the Raynaud's group, vasoconstriction was most marked during the late cold period (24.1 ± 21.2%), then late OR (26.6 ± 25.4%), then early cold (29.3 20.0%). For the control group, greatest vasoconstriction was as a response to a cognitive stressor, late MA (22.6 ± 25.3%) and early MA (26.5 ± 20.2%), then late cold challenge (27.2 ± 13.0%).

Right-hand mean relative constriction scores (percent of range) generally mimicked those for the left hand: Raynaud's patients showed lower overall percent scores, more stability of relative amplitudes across tasks, and more relative vasoconstriction to the early and late cold challenges. Standard deviations were again large for all mean group scores.

CONCLUSIONS

The finger temperature of Raynaud's patients as a group dropped in response to the cold stressors and remained supressed during the post-cold rest period. Controls were slightly more affected by emo-tional and cognitive stressors than by cold. Control subjects were

Table 4

	Rest	Early OR	Late OR	Early MA	Late MA	Rest	Early C	Late C	Rest

LEFT HAND -- PULSE WAVE AMPLITUDE (Percent of Range)

Raynaud's Diathesis

	Rest	Early OR	Late OR	Early MA	Late MA	Rest	Early C	Late C	Rest
X̄	38.9	29.9	26.6	32.0	32.2	40.6	29.3	24.3	37.4
SD	± 37.4	± 16.2	± 25.4	± 16.8	± 13.1	± 20.3	± 20.0	± 21.2	± 31.1

Control

	Rest	Early OR	Late OR	Early MA	Late MA	Rest	Early C	Late C	Rest
X̄	57.0	43.6	36.9	26.5	22.6	44.1	32.8	27.2	42.3
SD	± 20.0	± 21.7	± 22.2	± 20.2	± 25.3	± 25.2	± 15.3	± 13.0	± 21.1

RIGHT HAND -- PULSE WAVE AMPLITUDE (Percent of Range)

Raynaud's Diathesis

	Rest	Early OR	Late OR	Early MA	Late MA	Rest	Early C	Late C	Rest
X̄	38.99	37.75	35.47	37.77	37.77	42.35	37.58	34.13	39.81
SD	± 23.05	± 19.66	± 16.53	± 23.78	± 18.73	± 21.24	± 17.72	± 17.00	± 17.10

Control

	Rest	Early OR	Late OR	Early MA	Late MA	Rest	Early C	Late C	Rest
X̄	61.91	55.24	49.57	33.33	30.57	58.14	45.40	39.17	49.27
SD	± 18.86	± 21.10	± 16.22	± 22.98	± 21.87	± 13.43	± 22.89	± 17.26	± 23.60

Legend: See Legend of Table 1 for explanation of tasks.

also more likely to increase finger temperature to baseline values
during the post-cold rest period. These differences, however, were
not statistically significant above the P = 0.20 level, indicating
considerable overlap in the distributions.

Absolute pulse amplitudes were significantly lower in the
scleroderma patients, indicating either less blood flow in the
extremities or greater absorbance of infrared light due to the build
up of sclerodactylous or collagen tissue in the digit measures.

When using group statistical analysis, Raynaud's patients
across tasks were not clearly distinguishable from normal controls
on the measures of finger temperature and relative pulse amplitude.
Absolute pulse amplitudes were, however, clearly lower for the experimental group, especially for the scleroderma subgroup.
Together, these data may be interpreted to suggest that Raynaud's
patients, and especially scleroderma patients, suffer from
restricted peripheral capillary blood flow which only marginally
influences resting temperature responses and relative vasomotor
reactivity to most laboratory stressors. Thus, Raynaud's patients
respond to most non-cold stressors in a manner not too unlike our
normal controls.

In the case of the cold challenge, however, Raynaud's patients
typically showed lingering vasoconstriction between cold stimuli and
in the five minutes following the cold challenge. This effect was
most apparent in finger temperature measures and least evident in
the relative pulse amplitude measures.

These results are consistent with the self-reports of our
Raynaud's patients that their hands respond almost exclusively to
mild cold rather than to emotional or cognitive stressors. Only one
patient reported episodic vasospasms when emotionally stressed;
this exceptional patient had mild Raynaud's disease, not
scleroderma.

Overall, these results caution that the psychophysiological
profile does not discern scleroderma patients from normals using
only finger temperatures and relative blood flow measures. The profile does distinguish Raynaud's disease patients from normals,
however. Absolute finger blood flow measures combined with temperature recovery curves are most discriminative, particularly when
comparing degree of post-cold recovery. The outcome is particularly
surprising because 14 of our 15 Raynaud's patients did not respond
to the laboratory cold challenge with a true episodic peripheral
vasospastic attack. All patients did report the palmar cold stimulus to be very cold, even painful. Thus, the psychophysiological
differences in post-cold recovery tend to occur even in the absence
of the Raynaud's episode, confirming earlier observations in the
clinical literature (see Coffman and Davies, 1975).

PART II: TREATMENT ALTERNATES: PHARMACOLOGICAL, SURGICAL AND
          BIOBEHAVIORAL INTERVENTIONS

Nearly all current biomedical treatments assume that
vasospastic attacks in Raynaud's phenomenon are caused by excessive
sympathetic nervous system activity and/or vasomotor receptor
hypersensitivity. The final cause for acute capillary constriction
is viewed as some form of denervation-like hypersensitivity or
reflex hypersensitivity to endogenous vasoactive agents. This
assumption has led to the use of vasomotor drug therapy for mild
forms of the disease and sympathectomy for more severe cases.

MEDICO/SURGICAL TREATMENTS

The ideal prophylactic drug would specifically and uniquely
dilate the peripheral blood vessels. Unfortunately, available vaso-
dilator drugs appear to have non-specific effects on all blood
vessels of the body. Given systemically, these drugs produce their
largest effect on the larger vascular reservoirs so that systemic
drug therapy may in fact draw blood away from the extremities and
produce orthostatic hypotension.

Reserpine depletes norepinephrine, dopamine, and serotonin
from the brain and other tissues, presumably by interfering with
their storage. Reserpine also appears to produce a brief but direct
vasodilation independent of norepinephrine. Oral daily doses of as
little as 0.25-0.50 mg. have produced dramatic symptom reduction in
Raynaud's patients in as little as three weeks, although doses of
0.75-1.00 mg. are often necessary. Side effects, however, are
unpleasant, and the drug regimen must be reduced or stopped if signs
of nausea, fatigue, nightmares, or depression appear. Intra-
arterial Reserpine, once used to reduce pain and ulceration in
Raynaud's disease, appears to have variable effects and is not
effective in long-term therapy (Willerson et al., 1970).

Alphamethyldopa is a decarboxylase inhibitor which inter-
feres with both dopamine and serotonin synthesis. It is a powerful
anti-hypertensive agent. Typical effective doses in Raynaud's
patients are about 1.5 - 2.0 gms. per day. Its mode of action in
preventing vasospastic attacks is unknown, but it is presumed to be
due to depletion of norepinephrine. Not surprisingly, Alphamethyldopa has some minor side effects, such as lethargy, nausea, and
edema, as well as a potential for inducing postural hypotension and
helolytic anemia (Varadi & Lawrence, 1969).

Guanethidine in doses of 30-50 mgs. per day taken for
4 to 6 weeks appears to enhance peripheral blood flow in Raynaud's
patients. This drug has a mechanism of action thought to be similar
to that of Reserpine, but it is not well understood. Side effects
of postural hypotension, drowsiness, and impotence or retrograde

ejaculation makes it unsuitable for general use in vasospastic
diseases (Leroy, Downey & Cannon, 1971).

        Griseofulvin is a fungistatic antibiotic which appears to
have a direct dilatory action on vascular smooth muscle.
Griseofulvin continues to cause vasodilation in the presence of
ganglionic adrenergic, cholinergic and histaminic blocking agents.
Oral doses of 0.5-2.0 gms. per day have been reported to reduce
successfully vasospastic attacks in the majority of patients (Allen,
1971). This drug shares the major side effects of oral antibiotics,
including especially the problems of diarrhea and liver function
abnormalities.

        Uncontrolled positive clinical reports can also be found for
the use of estrogenic therapy for Raynaud's disease associated with
menopause. Talazoline and phenoxybenzamine have also been explored.
Propranolol is relatively contraindicated in Raynaud's phenomenon.

        Sympathectomy is almost always beneficial, at least
temporarily, for Raynaud's disease, but is contraindicated in the
presence of collagen disease (see Coffman and Davies, 1975;
Fairbairn, 1972). In the long run, sympathectomy may produce dener-
vation hypersensitivity in the peripheral vasomotor beds, making
vasoconstriction to circulating amines even more intense and prolonged (Guyton, 1971).

BIOFEEDBACK TREATMENT IN RAYNAUD'S DIATHESIS (See Table 5)

        Lisina (1958) was the first to report that normal subjects
could learn to control forearm blood flow if allowed to observe
their own plethysmographic readouts. Although a number of
intriguing experiments were performed to explore the phenomenon of
voluntary feedback-assisted blood flow, voluntary temperature
control was not examined until the early 1970s. Taub and Emurian
(1972) trained subjects to either increase or decrease hand temperature feedback training by showing that it could be incorporated
into migraine headache treatment programs.

        The application of clinical temperature biofeedback tech-
niques to Raynaud's disease phenomenon was first reported by Surwit
(1973). Using thermal biofeedback, a 21-year-old female was able to
increase her basal skin temperature (both hands) from 23°C to
26.6°C. Peper (1973), Jacobson et al. (1973), and Shapiro and
Schwartz (1972) were also successful in teaching subjects to raise
hand temperature or increase blood flow to an extremity. The latter
authors used a photoplethysmograph rather than temperature as their
feedback modality.

        Blanchard and Haynes (1975) treated one case of Raynaud's
disease with differential visual feedback for reducing the dif-

Table 5

AUTHORS	NUMBER OF PATIENTS	TREATMENT(S) USED	RESULTS	LENGTH OF FOLLOW-UP
Shapiro & Schwartz (1972)	1	Photoplethysmography of big toe.	Control of symptoms for 1 year.	None
Jacobson et al., (1973)	1	Differential biofeedback of temporal artery and finger temperature.	Much symptomatic improvement.	7-1/2 months
Peper (1973)	1	Differential biofeedback of temporal artery and finger temperatures.	Much improvement; basal skin temperature increased by 10°F.	None
Surwit (1973)	1	Biofeedback of digital temperature.	Temperature increased 3.6°C for 1 year.	No systematic data
Blanchard & Haynes (1975)	1	Differential biofeedback of hand and forehead temperatures.	Symptomatic improvement, basal hand temperature increased by 12°F.	7 months
May & Weber (1974)	8	Biofeedback of digital skin temperature.	Marked reduction of frequency of vasospastic episodes; all patients learned to warm hands.	None
Sedlacek (1977)	3	Thermal biofeedback & EMG feedback for relaxation.	All patients learned to warm hands.	None
Stephenson (1977)	2	Digital thermal biofeedback & EMG feedback from the frontalis.	Symptomatic remission; basal skin temperature increased by 10°F.	8-16 months
Freedman et al., (1978)	8	Digital thermal biofeedback.	Relief, but no subject was completely symptom free.	None
Surwit et al., (1978)	32	Biofeedback of skin temperature.	Reduction in frequency of vasospastic episodes; maintained normal skin temperature in 17°C.	None

ference between finger and forehead temperature. This case was ear-
marked by being the first patient treated solely by biofeedback.
These results were sufficiently favorable to encourage further
investigations in the treatment of Raynaud's patients with these
techniques. More recently, Freedman et al. (1978) systematically
replicated Blanchard and Haynes' study by employing only biofeedback
temperature training (i.e., without relaxation exercises) in the
treatment of eight persons suffering from primary and secondary
Raynaud's phenomenon. Interestingly, results showed that patients
with secondary Raynaud's phenomenon were more successful in raising
hand temperatures than patients with primary Raynaud's phenomenon
(presumably Raynaud's disease). However, all Raynaud's patients
were less successful in elevating finger temperature than were
normals.

Encouraging results were obtained by May and Weber (1977)
utilizing temperature feedback training for voluntary control of
finger skin temperature in eight cases of primary and secondary
Raynaud's disease. Contrary to expectations, Raynaud's patients
were found to be better temperature elevators than control subjects.
Secondary Raynaud's patients were again more successful in raising
finger temperature than primary Raynaud's patients (congruent with
Freedman et al.'s 1978 study). Moreover, the degree of symptomatic
improvement (i.e., the number of vasospastic episodes) was significantly correlated with success at temperature elevation.

Together, these anecdotal case reports and case studies
suggest that biofeedback techniques may be one modality of treatment
for Raynaud's diathesis and related vasodysregulatory disorders.
This conclusion awaits confirmation by large sample, controlled outcome studies comparing biofeedback with other treatments.

Surwit, Pilon and Fenton (1978), studied 32 female patients
afflicted with primary Raynaud's disease. There were four treatment
conditions: (1) autogenic training and skin temperature feedback in
the laboratory; (2) autogenic training alone in the laboratory; (3)
autogenic training instructions for home practice; and (4) skin temperature feedback plus autogenic instructions for home practice.
(Autogenic training uses a series of repeated verbal self-
suggestions to train patients in relaxation and stress-reduction).
Results revealed that all treatments were equally effective; subjects in all groups reported a diminution of vasospastic attacks in
frequency and in intensity. Furthermore, subjects were successful
in maintaining near normal levels of digital skin temperature in an
ambient temperature of 17°C during the cold stressor test.

Surwit et al. (1978) thus concluded that digital thermal
training biofeedback did not significantly improve the treatment
effect obtained from autogenic training alone. These data, however,
fail to evaluate whether biofeedback training per se (or in com-

bination with other modalities) is truly effective under optimal
training conditions. Thus, it is premature to rule out biofeedback
training as a biobehavioral technique in controlling vasospastic
episodes related to Raynaud's diathesis.

In support of the utilization of biofeedback training as a
viable alternative treatment for Raynaud's patients is Sedlacek's
(1977) treatment of three cases of Raynaud's disease. Thermal
training and frontalis EMG biofeedback were chosen as a potential
means of augmenting relaxation and relaxation-induced vasodilation,
which presumably increase peripheral temperature. Unfortunately,
patients were given autogenic instructions for home practice, so
success cannot be attributed solely to the biofeedback techniques.
Similarly, Stephenson (1977) employed deep muscle relaxation, autogenic training, and psychotherapy as adjuncts to pure frontalis EMG
feedback, therefore contaminating any clear-cut results.

It appears then, that clinical biofeedback training as a biobehavioral treatment holds promise, but there are some unresolved
issues concerning application and efficacy. One issue is whether
biobehavioral interventions would be more suitable for certain
subclasses of patients with vasomotor disorders. Surwit et al.
(1978) found that the revenge frequency and intensity of self-
reported vasospastic attacks during the autogenic/biofeedback
training period was significantly lower (between 1.2 to 1.8 attacks
per day) than before training (2.1 to 2.5 attacks per day).
Patients reported that they were able to maintain a decrease in
attacks when contacted post-treatment, but no data were provided
concerning the nature of the contact or the length of the follow-up.

The paucity of data is reflected in the lack of precision in
the diagnosis of Raynaud's disease versus Raynaud's phenomenon.
Many studies refer to Raynaud-like symptoms (Jacobson et al., 1973;
Peper, 1973). The diagnostic terminology has not been constant
(e.g., the patient in the Blanchard and Haynes study is referred to
both as a Raynaud's disease and Raynaud's phenomenon patient; see
also Freedman et al., 1978).

Voluntary hand temperature warming using biofeedback or other
biobehavioral techniques involves local vasodilation, but it is not
clear at what level such voluntary vasodilation occurs. It has been
suggested, for example, that a vasospastic Raynaud's attack may
involve an abnormal shunting of blood away from the skin
(arteriovenous anastomoses). If arteriovenous shunting is indeed
the major mechanism producing the attack, temperature biofeedback
could raise finger temperature by increasing flow through the shunt
without restoring capillary flow. Such shunting may have occurred
in one patient who continued to report pain even after her finger
temperature returned to normal (Surwit, 1973).

Early pilot studies in this laboratory with finger temperature biofeedback in three patients with Raynaud's disease have indicated that they can be taught to raise dominant hand finger temperature by 3° to 5^OC. One patient reported that she was able to prevent a vasospastic attack when it was anticipated (i.e., when getting something from the freezer, for example) and reverse an attack once begun. Thus, this patient was able to apply her learning in the laboratory as a therapeutic modality in the home situation.

SPECIFICITY OF TEMPERATURE BIOFEEDBACK TRAINING

Schwartz (1973) found that blood flow in a Raynaud's patient apparently increased at the site of the training thermistor, the toe, but did not increase in the contralateral site until it was specifically monitored. In other words, vasomotor self-control at one site did not spontaneously generalize to another site.

In contrast, two recent studies found evidence of situational generalization of temperature elevation. Taub (1977) found that Raynaud's subjects (n = 3) could not only be trained to elevate web-dorsum (hand) temperature (up to 10^OC in one subject), but could maintain the vasodilation effect at the same site without benefit of instrumented feedback in _cold_ environments. Sappington (1977) successfully trained a patient with systemic lupus erythematosus to raise finger temperature. The latency of the temperature increase progressively shortened across sessions, a phenomenon interpreted as situational generalization of the response. The increased laboratory hand temperature was also consistent with verbal reports of success outside the laboratory through home practice. Particularly interesting were her reports of maintaining elevated temperatures in _cold_ environments which previously elicited Raynaud's episodes.

In summary, localized temperature training alone does not appear to generalize to adjacent or contralateral skin sites without additional multi-site generalization training. However, situational generalization--i.e., from warm to cold environments--has been found, suggesting that a technique such as cold "inoculation" may itself enhance a multi-site generalized autonomic response of peripheral vasodilitation. Thus, while simple temperature training may yield a highly localized training response, exposure to previously noxious environments may establish a more generalized set of autonomic defenses against cold-induced vasoconstriction. We tested this hypothesis in the following experiment.

EXPERIMENT II: EFFECTS OF PROGRESSIVE COLD INOCULATION TRAINING ON
                 PERIPHERAL THERMAL REGULATION IN RAYNAUD'S PATIENTS

This experiment assessed the patients' physiological responses to localized cold before and after biofeedback treatment.

Treatment was divided into two phases: simple cutaneous temperature
elevation biofeedback training and biofeedback-assisted cold inoculation training. Patients received temperature biofeedback and cold
inoculation training for the left index finger. Temperatures of the
right and left index fingers were simultaneously monitored.

The first two weeks of the experiment were devoted to recording
symptoms in daily symptom log charts. At the same time, the
patients underwent the baseline psychophysiological stress evaluation outlined in Experiment I. They were then scheduled to come
three times per week for a minimum of 12 sessions of biofeedback and
cold inoculation training. After simple finger temperature elevation training, patients were assigned to commence cold inoculation
training.

Five patients volunteered for this study. Two scleroderma
patients could not complete the training due to illness. The
remaining three patients consisted of one scleroderma patient and
two Raynaud's disease patients. Patients were not allowed to participate if they exhibited any of the following: (a) functionally
disabling congestive heart failure; (b) severe intractable abdominal
pain, GI bleeding or diarrhea; (c) consumption of vasoactive compounds (e.g., Alphamethyldopa, Reserpine, Clonidine, Prazosine,
phenothiazines, Imipramine, etc.); (d) prior sympathectomy of upper
or lower extremities; or (e) functional disability--inability to
come to the clinic as required by the protocol.

Biofeedback training and testing was conducted in the experimental room of the Clinical Psychophysiology Service of the
Sepulveda VA Medical Center. An Autogenics 2000 Feedback
Thermometer was programmed for continuous or pulse-proportional
direct absolute cutaneous temperature feedback. The cold stimulus
for cold inoculation training was provided to the left palmar surface by recessing a thermoelectric cold plate (Thermoelectrics,
Model TCP-2) flush with the left arm of the chair. A thermistor was
implanted into the cold plate, so that temperature could be manually
regulated by the technician via a rheostat in an adjacent room.

Procedure

Upon entry into this experiment, all patients were provided
with a Symptom Daily Log Chart by the CPL staff. Patients were then
instructed in self-charting of their symptoms. During training,
they were also instructed to practice at home whatever cognitive
strategy produced cutaneous temperature elevation in the laboratory.

The experiment consisted of five components: (a) pretreatment
cold challenge; (b) voluntary cutaneous temperature elevation; (c)
biofeedback training; (d) cold inoculation training with biofeedback; and (e) post-treatment cold challenge.

Pre-Treatment Cold Challenge. The pre-treatment challenge was
part of the psychophysiological test described in detail in
Experiment I, Part II, A. In brief, following a 5-minute rest, the
cold plate was activated for 2-minute epochs, each punctuated by a
2-minute rest. Cold stimuli were sequentially reduced from 23.9°C
to 7.2°C over a 20-minute period. There was a final 5 minutes of
rest for measuring recovery.

Pre-Feedback Voluntary Temperature Elevation. In this initial,
training-like session each patient was required to sit quietly for
40 minutes, the length of the forthcoming biofeedback sessions.
Patients were instructed to attempt to warm their hands by any mental techniques available; no suggestions were given. The training
thermistor was placed on the dorsal interphalangeal surface of the
left index finger, distal to the left palmar cold plate. This
session was divided into five components: (a) stabilization (10
minutes), (b) elevation instruction (10 minutes), (c) rest 1 (5
minutes), (d) elevation instruction (10 minutes), and (e) rest 2 (5
minutes). As in the two training protocols, the experimenter was
present in the biofeedback room during rest 1 and rest 2.

Temperature Elevation Training Protocol. The dorsal surface of
the left index finger was arbitrarily selected as the thermal
biofeedback training site; the physical limitations of the laboratory dictated that the cold plate (used for cold inoculation
training) could only be set up for the left hand. The dorsal surface of the right index finger was additionally monitored. The dorsal surface was chosen to permit signal detection uncontaminated by
direct contact with the arm of the chair or the cold plate.

Each session was divided into five components: (a) stabilization, (b) biofeedback 1, (c) rest 1, (d) biofeedback 2, (e) rest 2.
Stabilization was defined as no net temperature change or a change
no greater than 0.5°C occurring in the last five minutes of quiet
rest. Usually, this criterion was met in 10 minutes. If a change
greater than 0.5°C did occur, an additional five-minute period of
quiet rest was permitted before commencing training.

During both the first and second biofeedback training phases,
patients received direct proportional temperature increase feedback.
In the initial session, the experimenter was present in the feedback
room and described to the patient some techniques which are commonly
utilized to elevate temperature. After the first session, the
patient was alone during biofeedback.

During the rest periods, the experimenter was always with
the patient in the feedback room. The time was used to discuss
the problems encountered during the preceding biofeedback phase and
to suggest any alternatives or modifications that would be useful in
reaching the treatment goal.

Patients were seated in the experimental chair facing a
10 unit 2 cm by 10 cm amber "light bar" (Coulbourn Instruments
H15-01 Bar Graph Display) placed on a table two meters away. An
adjustable 0-30 decibels auditory (tone) feedback was given through
enclosed stereo speakers mounted into the top of the experimental
chair.

Auditory and visual feedback was provided by linking the out-
puts of an Autogen 2000 Temperature Unit (output sensitivity set at
0.05 volts per degree Fahrenheit) to the inputs of a Coulbourn
Instrument audioamplifier speaker for direct frequency-proportional
audio feedback (10 to 1100 Hz over $\pm$ 0.68^{o}C). The Autogen 2000
output was also amplified through a Coulbourn Instruments invert-
offset amplifier/voltage-controlled amplifier combination
(programmed to square the output signal X0.1) to boost the signal
for visual feedback. Visual feedback was provided by a Coulbourn
Instruments 12-segment LED light bar, located two meters in front of
the patient. The change in a single LED reflected a temperature
change at the thermistor site of 0.043^{o}F. A 1°F increase would
illuminate all LEDs, at which point all LEDs would flash for one
second to signal the patient that the unit was being recalibrated to
bring the lights back on scale. Only the light bar was readjusted.
The reference temperature and the auditory tone were not readjusted
during training. During the first session, the experimenter
explained the feedback system to the patients to make sure that they
understood the signals.

Cold Inoculation Training Protocol. Cold inoculation training
consisted of exposing the patient's left palm to a given cold stimulus for a preset length of time (20, 40, 60, 20 seconds) while
receiving temperature biofeedback. To implement this, a cold plate
(Thermoelectrics) was recessed into the arm of the experimental
chair (left side). A thermistor was attached to the cold plate;
cold plate temperature was controlled by the experimenter via a
rheostat in the adjacent room.

The cold inoculation training session was divided into the
same 5 components: stabilization, biofeedback 1, rest 1, biofeedback 2, and rest 2. The stabilization and the two rest phases were
identical to that of the temperature elevation training protocol.
At least one of the biofeedback phases was devoted to cold
inoculation. If the patient's left-hand temperature was 29°C or
greater during stabilization, cold inoculation was presented during
both biofeedback 1 and biofeedback 2. In the event that left-hand
temperature was below 29°C, training reverted to simple temperature
elevation without cold stimuli during the first biofeedback component and cold inoculation training only during the second biofeedback component.

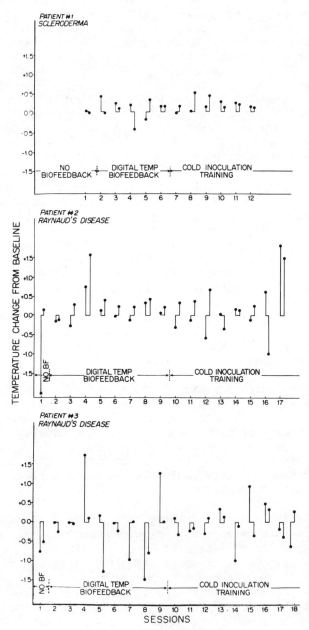

Figure 1(a) Digital temperature biofeedback training and cold inoculation training: Temperature change from baseline.

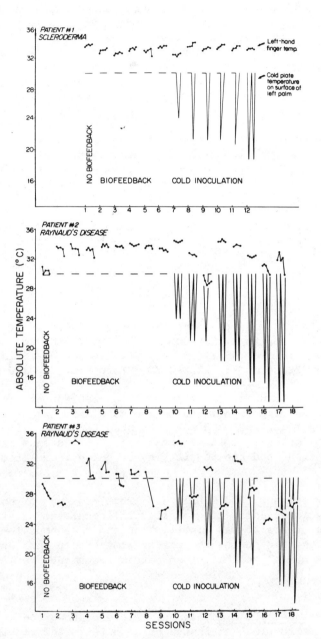

Figure 1(b)   Biofeedback training and cold inoculation training:
Absolute temperature (°C).

Patients entered cold inoculation following at least six
sessions of simple biofeedback training. Patient 1, with scleroderma, began cold inoculation training on session 7. Patients 2 and
3 were both afflicted with Raynaud's disease, and were of similar
ages, backgrounds, and motivations for cold inoculation. Their
responses to simple biofeedback training were, however, opposite.
Patient 2 rapidly demonstrated hand warming, while Patient 3 exhibited variable elevation over sessions (see Figure 1). Since par-
ticipation was limited to 18 sessions, we elected to expose both
patients to cold inoculation in session 10. This procedure matched
biofeedback and cold inoculation treatments for both patients at two
disparate levels of performance and allowed some inferences about
the role of early success in biofeedback upon subsequent success in
cold inoculation.

The patient was instructed to increase left-hand temperature
or at least to maintain warmth using the biofeedback skills already
acquired. She was never informed of the exact moment the cold plate
would be turned on. She was, however, informed what the plate temperature would be and the length of time the cold stimulus would
remain on.

Cold stimuli were presented in the following order: 23.9°C
(75°F) for 20, 40, 60, 120 seconds; 21.1°C (70°F) for 20, 40, 60,
120 seconds; 18.3°C (65°F) for 40, 60, 120 seconds; 15.6°C (60°F)
for 40, 60, 120 seconds; 12.8°C (55°F) for 40, 60, 120 seconds.

In most instances, the time interval between two cold stimuli
was the length of presentation of the cold stimulus, ± 20 seconds.
For example, if 23.9°C cold was presented for a duration of 60
seconds, the inter-stimuli interval was 40-80 seconds. In this
way, the patient had the possibility of being inoculated 50% of the
time.

Post-Treatment Cold Challenge. This test was given to assess
whether the intervening program of cold inoculation training would
improve resistance to vasoconstriction and cutaneous temperature
decrement observed during the pre-treatment cold challenge. This
test was identical to that given before treatment.

RESULTS

Pre-Treatment Cold Challenge. Table 6 shows the effects of the
left palmar cold plate challenge on both left- and right-hand finger
temperatures and pulse amplitudes for Patients 1, 2, and 3. To
simplify comparisons, results are given as the means and standard
deviations for rest 1 (10 minutes), early cold, from 29.4 to 18.3°C,
(10 minutes), late cold, from 12.8 to 7.2°C (10 minutes) and rest 2
(5 minutes).

Table 6

LEFT-HAND TEMPERATURES (Centigrade)

	Rest I	Early Cold	Late Cold	Rest II
Patient 1				
PRE	31.93±0.25	32.14±0.14	31.45±0.46	30.5±0.06
POST	32.21±0.39	32.82±0.07	32.74±0.27	33.02±0.11
Patient 2				
PRE	30.39±0.18	28.69±0.84	27.49±0.34	27.46±0.68
POST	30.42±0.32	29.01±0.32	29.43±0.79	29.06±0.52
Patient 3				
PRE	30.88±0.12	29.62±0.6	28.75±0.39	28.75±1.57
POST	26.16±0.07	24.94±0.14	25.76±0.34	26.54±0.18

LEFT-HAND PULSE (mV-S)

	Rest I	Early Cold	Late Cold	Rest II
Patient 1				
PRE	9.78±0.92	7.89±1.38	5.84±1.27	7.7±3.89
POST	12.01±1.65	12.25±1.82	10.16±1.94	11.12±0.81
Patient 2				
PRE	25.05±3.89	10.06±2.02	18.74±14.59	48.96±5.92
POST	17.07±6.61	17.51±16.41	12.11±5.84	18.62±2.82
Patient 3				
PRE	23.23±3.08	12.36±5.47	5.15±4.88	45.1±8.33
POST	9.58±5.55	8.26±3.64	12.1±6.03	24.93±14.45

RIGHT-HAND TEMPERATURES (Centigrade)

	Rest I	Early Cold	Late Cold	Rest II
Patient 1				
PRE	34.2±.014	33.83±0.05	33.31±0.24	33.36±0.15
POST	33.58±0.13	33.83±0.05	33.98±0.1	34.06±0.06
Patient 2				
PRE	31.67±0.15	29.55±0.84	28.19±0.44	30.24±0.78
POST	31.67±0.19	30.5±0.81	31.51±0.83	32.84±0.73
Patient 3				
PRE	31.64±0.27	29.93±0.37	29.93±0.6	31.46±0.69
POST	26.68±0.17	25.94±0.22	26.35±0.11	26.78±0.21

RIGHT-HAND PULSE (mV-S)

	Rest I	Early Cold	Late Cold	Rest II
Patient 1				
PRE	23.65±3.17	24.88±3.84	15.06±2.58	17.07±4.08
POST	16.75±3.52	15.48±3.26	14.52±3.38	11.88±1.55
Patient 2				
PRE	28.53±4.14	18.65±4.79	23.4±7.56	34.14±2.93
POST	21.57±1.35	15.46±7.76	16.33±5.41	23.77±5.53
Patient 3				
PRE	41.83±8.39	30.62±7.7	29.08±11.18	47.42±11.12
POST	10.49±7.25	11.46±3.91	18.78±7.28	25.03±10.84

An individual analysis of these three pre-treatment cold test profiles generally reflects those of the Raynaud's patients as a group in Experiment I. Patient 1, with scleroderma, remained above 30°C throughout testing. She showed a small but negligible temperature response to the first cold challenge, in part related to apparent vasoconstriction (finger pulse amplitudes below 10 mV-sec in the left hand). Her non-stressed right hand was warmer (about 34°C) and more dilated (about 23 mV-sec) and showed relatively more temperature decrease and vasoconstriction than the left hand in response to the cold stimulus.

Patients 2 and 3, both with Raynaud's disease, showed a drop from 30°C during rest to approximately 27-28°C during late cold, a decrease sustained during the second rest period. Digital pulse amplitudes for both Raynaud's patients were within normal range (about 23-25 mV-sec), but were reduced by 20 to 80% during late cold and dilated by more than 200% (45 to 48 mV-sec) during the second rest period. Thus, in spite of the lower cutaneous temperature, the two Raynaud's patients demonstrated a greater range of vasomotor responsivity than the scleroderma patient.

Digital Temperature Biofeedback Training. These results are summarized in Figure 1.

For Patient 1, relative temperatures increased in seven of 10 10-minute biofeedback components (sessions 2-6) by at least 0.20°C. For Patient 2, 11 of 16 components were increased across biofeedback sessions. For Patient 3, only 9 of 16 components were increased, and 6 of those 9 showed increases of less than 0.20°C. Patient 3 also exhibited wide session-to-session absolute temperature variability, ranging from 34.7°C in session 3 to 24.2°C in session 9.

Figure 1 shows the session-by-session effects of the cold inoculation training procedure. For Patient 1, left-hand finger temperature remained elevated more than 0.20°C above resting baseline in 10 or 12 biofeedback components, less than 0.20°C in one segment, and decreased less than 0.20°C in another segment. Cold inoculation stimuli failed to reduce finger temperature, even at a cold plate temperature of 18.3°C. This patient was exposed to seven cold inoculation components, averaging five 20-120 second stimuli per component, for a total of 24 cold stimulus presentations.

For Patient 2, temperatures were elevated 0.20°C or more in seven of 16 components, less than 0.20°C in three components, and declined in six components. She received a total of 75 cold stimuli, 15 of which were at 12.8°C (55°F). For Patient 3, temperatures were elevated above 0.20°C in three of 14, and decreased in 10 of 14 segments. During session 15, cold stimuli were not presented; finger temperature increased in both non-cold biofeedback

components. She received 65 cold stimulus presentations. Her absolute baseline finger temperatures varied widely, ranging from 35.3°C
in session 10 to 25.2°C in session 16.

Post-Treatment Cold Challenge. These data are shown in Table
6. For patient 1, left-hand cold challenge temperatures following
successful cold inoculation training remained elevated and relatively resistant to cold. This cold-resistive effect was also
reflected in left-hand finger pulse amplitudes, which showed 20 to
80% more vasodilation across the cold periods.

Similar treatment effects were found for Patient 2. Compared
with the pre-treatment cold challenge when left-hand finger temperature dropped almost 3°C, the post-treatment cold challenge
drop was only 1°C. Interestingly, mean left hand pulse amplitudes
during cold challenge were generally lower post-treatment (12-18
mV-sec) than before treatment (10-48 mV-sec).

Patient 3 showed some evidence of acquiring consistent vasomotor self-control skills during training. When given the cold
challenge following training, left-hand finger temperature remained
2 to 5°C lower than on the initial pre-training cold challenge.
Although her finger temperature was low, she was able to elevate her
temperature more than 1°C. Left-hand pulse amplitudes were similarly depressed until the post-cold rest period, when she
experienced digital vasodilation.

These three cases illustrate the wide range of individual
psychophysiological patterns and response acquisition curves typical
of the 11 Raynaud's patients referred to us for treatment over the
last three years. The clinical biofeedback training protocol presented here was time- and session-limited, which likely contributed
to the apparent failure of Patient 3 to demonstrate any vasomotor
self-regulation. Additional simple thermal feedback and perhaps
forearm EMG feedback to criterion would be recommended for this
patient. However, Patient 3 also had less opportunity for consistent home practice at any stage of training, unlike our other
patients who enthusiastically maintained home practice.

Subjective reports of Raynaud's episodes showed no relationship to training. However, training occurred during the warm
California summer when episodes are typically reduced to no more
than one or two per week. At three and six month follow-up, phone
interviews indicated reduced intensity of episodes for the scleroderma patient and increased cold tolerance for the successful
Raynaud's patient. Extreme temperature drops continued to elicit
Raynaud's episodes, but normal activities such as shopping in the
freezer section of a supermarket and playing night tennis by the
ocean were more easily tolerated by the two successful patients.

We are encouraged that the cold challenge data reliably predicted which patients benefited from the training program. However,
until larger samples, longer follow-ups, and placebo-control procedures are instituted, the relative efficacy of cold inoculation
training over simple biofeedback training remains unknown. We hope
that other laboratories will systematically replicate our procedure.
In the interim, we have been asked to give our clinical opinions
about choosing patients and training protocols most likely to yield
successful cold inoculation training.

INFLUENTIAL CLINICAL FACTORS IN TREATMENT OUTCOME

Who is a good candidate for biobehavioral treatment? Not
everyone will respond successfully to a treatment, no matter how
well designed. Here are some helpful guidelines we have evolved to
select Raynaud's patients who would benefit from biofeedback.

First, the psychophysiological stress battery can be used to
assess the extent of peripheral vascular pathophysiology. Should
the patient show little or no responsivity to either thermal or
emotional stress, prognosis is not hopeful. These patients exhibit profound vascular deterioration attenuating the physiological
mechanisms fundamental to cold resistance.

Second, the patient must be ambulatory. That is, if biofeedback treatment is to be effective, the patient must be capable of
coming to the office over a long period of time.

Third, the patient must be motivated. Personality characteristics may often be a helpful guide to assess the manner in which
the patient will respond to therapy. Generally, a person with
either rigid or hysterical personality traits will not be responsive
to a psychologically-based treatment modality. The hysterical
patient tends to be very enthused initially, but interest may wane
rapidly. The rigid patient, on the other hand, tends to be reti-
cent about the therapeutic value of biofeedback, but can sometimes
be swayed to acceptance. One of our patients, for example, was
diverted from her skeptical stance and began experiencing success
when she discovered that her son, a physician, was enthused about
biofeedback treatment. Thus, belief in the therapeutic technique is
essential for successful treatment. Reading an article about
biofeedback or talking to a former successful patient can be useful
in converting resistance to cooperation.

During the pre-treatment interview, the health professional
would do well to get information on the family dynamics pertaining
to coping mechanisms and secondary gains which likely maintain the
illness pattern. Some Raynaud's patients derive excessive sympathy
and attention from their illness, which may need to be dealt with in
psychotherapy, before biofeedback is attempted.

Fear of death and fear of disability are over-riding concerns in almost all of our scleroderma patients. Biofeedback training is often beneficial because even partial success can give the patient the feeling of more control over his illness and over his life. This tends to lessen his anxiety and perhaps alternate peripheral vasospasms mediated by catecholamines.

The next question which concerns the therapist is the mechanics of biofeedback treatment: how does one go about training the patient?

The biofeedback equipment itself must be sophisticated enough to measure fairly weak signals (pulse amplitude) and low temperatures. As Raynaud's phenomenon is defined as poor peripheral circulation, the photoplethysmographic signal must often be maximally amplified. It was a common occurrence in our laboratory to set the Coulbourn Instruments Pulse Monitor module to 10.0 (1.0-10.0 range). Similarly, it is a necessity to set the temperature feedback at maximum sensitivity so that the patient is able to see small changes. We recommend using a sensitivity of $1^{\circ} \pm 1$ Volt. If the biofeedback machine is not sensitive enough, it will not register small changes and the patient will tend to get discouraged.

Training the patient to augment finger temperature through biofeedback can be accomplished with or without adjunctive techniques. Temperature biofeedback may be used alone in conjunction with autogenic training, hypnosis, or guided imagery. In our laboratory, we emphasize adjunctive training-guided imagery. We also use a coach-trainee model, whereby the patient is said to be in physical conditioning for an Olympic temperature training program. The therapist "coaches" or guides him, utilizing mental imagery.

The choice of imagery to present to the patient is crucial. The therapist should first interview the patient pertaining to his hobbies and fantasies. The common image of visualizing oneself laying down on a beach with the sun warming the body is less than ideal if the subject dislikes the beach or cannot go out in the sun, as with the lupus erythematosus patient. Therefore, we advise finding some mental pictures that are tailored for each individual. For example, one of our patients warmed her finger temperature when she visualized re-decorating her house, another when playing a vigorous game of tennis.

CONCLUSION

Current medical treatments have not always been effective in Raynaud's disease/phenomenon. Thermal biofeedback may have clinical utility, but controlled studies of its efficacy compared to current medical treatments are lacking. Placebo and other psychological factors remain unevaluated.

Recent major reviews have questioned whether clinical biofeedback procedures are more efficacious than simple relaxation procedures based upon progressive relaxation, autogenic training, or meditational practices such as transcendental meditation (see Torler-Benlolo, 1978; Blanchard, 1978).

While the evidence is not yet complete for Raynaud's phenomenon, these conclusions concerning biofeedback versus relaxation for other disorders (headache and essential hypertension) may be premature. The majority of published clinical biofeedback procedures have attempted to train subjects to mimic physiological characteristics of a presumed low-arousal (i.e., relaxation) state. Therefore, it is not surprising that biofeedback protocols derived from stress-reduction procedures may yield clinical results similar to those for simple relaxation procedures.

Alternatives to relaxation-based biofeedback protocols have received no systematic evaluation in Raynaud's phenomenon. Unidirectional changes in finger temperature elevation support both passive relaxation and active learning models. Stronger support for specificity of the learning model may come from demonstration of voluntary control in the physiological responses during cold challenge testing. Successful training to resist cold-induced vasospasms would be strong evidence favoring a specific utilization of contingent biofeedback technology over and above its putative role in augmenting (or mimicking) non-specific relaxation. While the case studies presented here have yielded results consistent with improved performance following cold inoculation training, the efficacy, validity and reliability of such training remains to be compared directly to that for relaxation and simple biofeedback training.

In summary, thermal biofeedback may have clinical utility in Raynaud's diathesis. Controlled studies of its efficacy are few. Placebo and other psychological factors remain unevaluated. Cold inoculation training remains to be directly compared with other biobehavioral treatments.

ACKNOWLEDGEMENTS

We thank the VA Research Service and Dr. William H. Rickles for their support in this project. We acknowledge Deborah Rangel and Dr. Ken Tashiki in data analysis, and Dr. Thomas Sturm for technical assistance. Drs. Daniel Furst and Philip Clements of the UCLA Rheumatology Service screened, referred, and provided medical assistance to our patients. To our patients, we offer special thanks.

REFERENCES

Allen, B. R. Griseofulvin in Raynaud's phenomenon. Lancet,
 1971, 2, 840-841.

Birostingl, M. The Raynaud syndrome. Post Medical Journal,
 1971, 47, 1297.

Blair, A., Coller, F. A., & Conner, G. B. Raynaud's disease:
 A study of criteria for prognosis. Surgery, 1951, 29,
 387.

Blanchard, E. B. A data-based review of biofeedback, In
 Controversy in psychiatry. New York: MacMillan, 1978.

Blanchard, E. B., & Haynes, M. R. Biofeedback treatment in a
 case of Raynaud's disease. Journal of Behavior Therapy
 and Experimental Psychiatry, 1975, 6, 230-234.

Canon, P. J., Hassel, M., & Case, D. B., Casarella, W.J.,
 Sommers, S. C. & LeRoy, E. C. The relationship of
 hypertension and renal failure in scleroderma
 (progressive systemic sclerosis) to structural and functional abnormalities of the renal cortical circulation.
 Medicine, 1975, 53, (1).

Coffman, J. D., & Davies, W. T. Vasospastic diseases: a
 review. Progress in Cardiovascular Diseases, 1975, 18,
 123-146.

Davis, J., Furst, D., Clements, P., Chopra, S. K.,
 Theofilopoulos, A. N., & Paulus, H. E. Abnormalities of
 pulmonary, vascular, dynamics, and inflammation in early
 progressive systemic sclerosis. Arthritis and
 Rheumatism, 1979, 22, 604.

DeTakats, G., & Fowler, E. F. Raynaud's phenomenon. Journal of
 the American Medical Association, 1962, 179, 99-106.

Downey, J. A., & Frewin, D. B. The effect of cold on blood
 flow in the hands of patients with Raynaud's phenomenon.
 Clinical Science, 1973, 44, 279.

Fairbairn, J. F., Juergens, J. L., & Spittell, J. S., Jr.
 (Eds.). Allen-Barker-Hines peripheral vascular diseases
 (4th ed.). Philadelphia: W. B. Saunders, 1972.

Fordyce, W. E. Behavior methods for chronic pain and illness.
 St. Louis, MO: Mosby, 1976.

Freedman, R., Lynn, S. J., & Ianni, P. Biofeedback treatment of
 Raynaud's phenomenon. Proceedings from the 9th Annual
 Meeting of the Biofeedback Society of America.
 Albuquerque, NM, March 3-7, 1978, 83-84.

Fries, J. F. Clinical significance of Raynaud's phenomenon.
 Medical Digest, 1967, June, 15-20.

Fries, J., & Medsgar, W. Preliminary criteria for progressive
 systemic sclerosis. American Rheumatism Association,
 1978, 21, 712.

Gifford, R. W., Jr., & Hines, E. A., Jr. Raynaud's disease
 among women and girls. Circulation, 1957, 16, 1012.

Graham, D. T. Cutaneous vascular reactions in Raynaud's
       disease and its states of hostility, anxiety and
       depression. Psychosomatic Medicine, 1955, 17, 200-204.
Graham, D. T., Stein, J. A., & Winokin, G. Experimental
       investigation of the specificity of the attitude
       hypothesis in psychosomatic disease. Psychosomatic
       Medicine, 1958, 20, 446-457.
Guyton, A. Textbook of medical physiology. Philadelphia:
       W.B. Saunders, 1971.
Herzog, P., Clements, P. J., Roberts, N. K., Furst, D. E.,
       Johnson, C. E., & Feig, S. A. Case report: progressive
       systemic sclerosis-like syndrome following bone marrow
       transplantation. Clinical, immunologic, and pathologic
       findings. Journal of Rheumatology, 1980, 7, 56-64.
Jacobson, A. M., Hackett, T. P., Surman, O. S., & Silverberg,
       E. L. Raynaud's phenomenon. Treatment with hypnotic
       and operant technique. Journal of the American Medical
       Association, 1973, 225, (7), 739-740.
Jamieson, G. G., Ludbrook, J., & Wilson, A. Cold hypersensitiv-
       ity in Raynaud's phenomenon. Circulation, 1971, 44,
       254.
Kolvachik, M. T., Guggenheim, S. J., & Silverman, M. H. The
       kidney in progressive systemic sclerosis. Annuals of
       International Medicine, 1978, 89, 881-887.
Kontos, H. A., & Wasserman, A. J. Effect of reserpine in
       Raynaud's phenomenon. Circulation, 1969, 39, 259.
LeRoy, E. C., Downey, J. A., & Cannon, P. J. Skin capillary
       blood flow in scleroderma. The Journal of Clinical
       Investigation, 1971, 50, 930-939.
May, D. S., & Weber, C. A. Temperature feedback training for
       symptom reduction in primary and secondary Raynaud's
       disease. Biofeedback and Self-Regulation (Abstract),
       1977, 2 (3), 317.
Mendlowitz, N., & Naftchi, N. The digital circulation in
       Raynaud's disease. American Journal of Cardiology,
       1959, 4, 580.
Millet, J. A. Psychoanalytic psychotherapy in Raynaud's
       disease. Psychosomatic Medicine, 1956, 13 (6), 492-505.
Millet, J. A., Lief, H., & Mittleman, B. Raynaud's disease:
       psychogenic factors and psychotherapy. Psychosomatic
       Medicine, 1953, 15, 61.
Mittleman, B., & Wolff, H. G. Affective states and skin
       temperature. Psychosomatic Medicine, 1939, 1, 271.
Mittleman, B., & Wolff, H. G. Emotions and skin temperature:
       Observations on patients during psychotherapeutic
       (psychoanalytic) interviews. Psychosomatic Medicine,
       1943, 5, 211.
Mufson, I. The mechanism and treatment of Raynaud's disease:
       a psychosomatic disturbance. Annals of Internal
       Medicine, 1944, 20, 228.

Mufson, I. An etiology of scleroderma. Annals of Internal Medicine, 1953, 39, 1219.

Peacock, J. H. Peripheral venous blood concentration of epinephrine and norepinephrine in primary Raynaud's disease. Circulation Research, 1959, 7, 821.

Peper, E. Frontiers of clinical feedback, In Seminars in psychiatry. New York: Grune and Stratton, Vol. 5, 1973.

Pringle, R., Walder, D. M., & Weaver, J. P. Blood viscosity and Raynaud's disease. Lancet, 1965, 1, 1086.

Robinson, P. W., & Foster, D. F. Experimental psychology: A small-n approach. New York: Harper and Row, 1979.

Sapira, J. D., Rodnan, G. P., Scheib, E. T., Klaniecki, T., & Rizk, M. Studies of endogenous catecholamines in patients with Raynaud's phenomenon secondary to progressive systemic sclerosis (scleroderma). American Journal of Medicine, 1972, 52, 330.

Sappington, J. T. Operant conditioning of peripheral vaso-dilation in Raynaud's disease: a case study. Annual Meeting of the Southeastern Psychological Association, 1977.

Schwartz, G. E. Biofeedback as therapy: Some theoretical and practical issues. American Psychologist, 1973, 28, (8), 666-673.

Sedlacek, K. EMG and thermal feedback as a treatment for Raynaud's disease. Biofeedback and Self-Regulation (Abstract), 1977, 2 (3), 318.

Shapiro, D., & Schwartz, G. E. Biofeedback and visceral learning: Clinical applications. Seminars in Psychiatry, 1972, 4, 171-181.

Spittell, J. A. Raynaud's phenomenon and allied vasospastic conditions. In J. A. Spittell et al., Peripheral vascular diseases. Philadelphia: W. B. Saunders, 1974.

Stephenson, N. E. Two cases of successful treatment of Raynaud's disease with relaxation and biofeedback training and supportive psychotherapy. Biofeedback and Self-Regulation (Abstract), 1977, 2, 318-319.

Sternbach, R. A. Pain patients: Traits and treatment. New York: Academic Press, 1974.

Surwit, R. S. Biofeedback: A possible treatment for Raynaud's disease. In L. Birk (Ed.), Biofeedback: Behavioral medicine. New York: Grune & Stratton, 1973.

Surwit, R. S., Pilon, R. N., & Fenton, C. H. Behavioral treatment of Raynaud's disease. Journal of Behavioral Medicine, 1978, 1 (3), 323-335.

Tarler-Benlolo, L. The role of relaxation in biofeedback training: A critical review of the literature. Psychological Bulletin, 1978, 85 (4), 727-755.

Taub, E. Self-regulation of human tissue temperature. In
    G. E. Schwartz & J. Beatty (Eds.), <u>Biofeedback theory</u>
    <u>and research</u>, New York: Academic Press, 1977.
Taub, E., & Emurian, C. S. Autoregulation of skin temperature
    using a variable intensity feedback light. Paper pre-
    sented at the Second Annual Meeting of the Biofeedback
    Research Society, 1972.
Varadi, D. P., & Lawrence, A. M. Suppression of Raynaud's
    phenomenon by methyldopa. <u>Archives of Internal</u>
    <u>Medicine</u>, 1969, <u>124</u>, 13.
Velayos, E. E., Robinson, H., Porcuincula, F. U., & Masi, A.
    Clinical correlation analysis of 137 patients with
    Raynaud's phenomenon. <u>American Journal of Medical</u>
    <u>Science</u>, 1971, <u>262</u>, 347-356.
Willerson, J. T., Thompson, R. H., & Hookmen, P. Reserpine in
    Raynaud's disease and phenomenon. <u>Annals of Internal</u>
    <u>Medicine</u>, 1970, <u>72</u>, 17.

LIST OF CONTRIBUTORS

Muriel T. Belanger, M. A.
Psychology Department
Laval University
Quebec, Canada

Dr. Eleanor Criswell
Executive Director
Biofeedback Society of California
c/o Psychology Department
Sonoma State University
Rohnert Park, CA 94928

Dr. Bernard Engel
Chief, Laboratory of Behavioral Science
Gerontology Research Center
Baltimore City Hospitals
Baltimore, MD 21224

Dr. David S. Gans
Medical Director
Sandweiss Biofeedback Institute
9730 Wilshire Boulevard, #205
Beverly Hills, CA 90212

Dr. Judith Green
Aims Biofeedback Institute
Aims Community College
P.O. 69
Greeley, CO 80632

Dr. Robert N. Grove
Clinical Psychophysiology
Veteran's Hospital, Sepulveda
Sepulveda, CA 91343

Dr. David Jacobs
Director
Biofeedback Institute of
   San Diego
2850 Sixth Avenue
San Diego, CA 92103

Dr. Lee Kudrow
Director
California Medical Clinic
   for Headache, Inc.
16542 Ventura Boulevard
Encino, CA 91436

Dr. Robert Miller
Assistant Clinical
   Professor
U.C.L.A. School of
   Medicine
7301 Medical Center Drive
Canoga Park, CA 91307

Dr. William H. Rickles
1100 Glendon Avenue, #1449
Los Angeles, CA 90024

233

Jack H. Sandweiss, M. A.
Director
Sandweiss Biofeedback
  Institute
9730 Wilshire Boulevard
  #205
Beverly Hills, CA 90212

Dr. Brien L. Tiep
Director of Pulmonary
  Rehabilitation
City of Hope Medical Center
Duarte, CA 91010

Dr. Steven L. Wolf
Associate Professor
Department of Rehabilitation
  Medicine
Center for Rehabilitation
  Medicine
1441 Clifton Road N.E.
Atlanta, GA 30322

INDEX